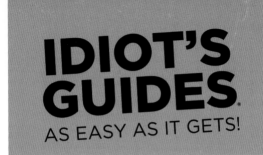

IDIOT'S GUIDES.

AS EASY AS IT GETS!

Reflexology

by Bill Flocco

ALPHA

A member of Penguin Group (USA) Inc.

ALPHA BOOKS

Published by Penguin Group (USA) Inc.

Penguin Group (USA) Inc., 375 Hudson Street, New York, New York 10014, USA • Penguin Group (Canada), 90 Eglinton Avenue East, Suite 700, Toronto, Ontario M4P 2Y3, Canada (a division of Pearson Penguin Canada Inc.) • Penguin Books Ltd., 80 Strand, London WC2R 0RL, England • Penguin Ireland, 25 St. Stephen's Green, Dublin 2, Ireland (a division of Penguin Books Ltd.) • Penguin Group (Australia), 250 Camberwell Road, Camberwell, Victoria 3124, Australia (a division of Pearson Australia Group Pty. Ltd.) • Penguin Books India Pvt. Ltd., 11 Community Centre, Panchsheel Park, New Delhi—110 017, India • Penguin Group (NZ), 67 Apollo Drive, Rosedale, North Shore, Auckland 1311, New Zealand (a division of Pearson New Zealand Ltd.) • Penguin Books (South Africa) (Pty.) Ltd., 24 Sturdee Avenue, Rosebank, Johannesburg 2196, South Africa • Penguin Books Ltd., Registered Offices: 80 Strand, London WC2R 0RL, England

International Standard Book Number: 978-1-61564-654-8
Library of Congress Catalog Card Number: 2014941125

16 15 14   8 7 6 5 4 3 2 1

Interpretation of the printing code: The rightmost number of the first series of numbers is the year of the book's printing; the rightmost number of the second series of numbers is the number of the book's printing. For example, a printing code of 14-1 shows that the first printing occurred in 2014.

Note: This publication contains the opinions and ideas of its author. It is intended to provide helpful and informative material on the subject matter covered. It is sold with the understanding that the author and publisher are not engaged in rendering professional services in the book. If the reader requires personal assistance or advice, a competent professional should be consulted. The author and publisher specifically disclaim any responsibility for any liability, loss, or risk, personal or otherwise, which is incurred as a consequence, directly or indirectly, of the use and application of any of the contents of this book.

Most Alpha books are available at special quantity discounts for bulk purchases for sales promotions, premiums, fund-raising, or educational use. Special books, or book excerpts, can also be created to fit specific needs. For details, write: Special Markets, Alpha Books, 375 Hudson Street, New York, NY 10014.

Trademarks: All terms mentioned in this book that are known to be or are suspected of being trademarks or service marks have been appropriately capitalized. Alpha Books and Penguin Group (USA) Inc. cannot attest to the accuracy of this information. Use of a term in this book should not be regarded as affecting the validity of any trademark or service mark.

The foot, hand, and ear reflexology maps used in this book are based on Bill Flocco's reflexology charts.

Publisher: **Mike Sanders**

Senior Production Editor: **Janette Lynn**

Executive Managing Editor: **Billy Fields**

Indexer: **Angie Bess Martin**

Development Editorial Supervisor: **Christy Wagner**

Layout: **Ayanna Lacey**

Design Supervisor: **William Thomas**

Proofreader: **Cate Schwenk**

Contents

Part 6   Reflexology for the Ears   119

Part 7   Reflexology for Everyone   137

Part 8   Reflexology for Relief   161

Introduction

An elderly widow's headache goes away. A young construction worker finds relief from agonizing back pain. A teen receives dramatic relief from her unfortunate food poisoning. A middle-age man goes from getting up six times a night to use the restroom to only once a night—in a single day. What do these people all have in common? Reflexology.

These stories are not unusual. Millions of people all over the world have experienced similar results, and hundreds of studies validate the wide range of benefits foot, hand, and ear reflexology provides.

My journey into reflexology started in 1981. Within 6 months of learning foot reflexology, I discovered hand reflexology. About that same time, two physicians exposed me to the medical approach of working with the map of the body on the outer ear. By the end of 1982, I was working with foot, hand, and ear reflexology. Little did I know that doing so would profoundly change my life.

While working with all three areas, it didn't take me long to realize that reflexing the feet is better for relief in certain parts and functions of the body, working the hands is best for other parts and functions, and focusing on the ears is more beneficial for other areas. I also found that working with all three—feet, hands, and ears—during the same reflexology session yields far greater benefits than working with just one area alone.

Think back over the past 6 months to health complaints you, your family, or your friends might have experienced, from allergies and headaches, to back pain, heartburn, and motion sickness, to toothaches and urinary tract infections. Now imagine giving yourself or those you care for safe, caring, nurturing touch through reflexology, knowing just where and how to work on the feet, hands, and ears for relief. Reflexology also can provide deep relaxation, stress reduction, and prevention of future health problems. More than anything, reflexology is a proactive way of ensuring you don't succumb to the tensions and pressures of life; of reducing, minimizing, or eliminating health problems when they do manifest; and of maintaining good, vibrant health.

I've made this book as easy to use as possible. In the following pages, you learn about reflexology, its benefits, and how to perform the reflexing techniques correctly. I've also included a compendium of ailments, issues, and other conditions reflexology can help reduce or relieve. Each section explains—with clear and easy-to-understand text instructions along with illustrative color photos showing just what moves to make on the feet, hands, and ears—how to best use reflexology for relief.

You are on the verge of a magnificent adventure into the world of reflexology. This book will serve you well on your journey.

Acknowledgments

I would like to express heartfelt love and gratitude to my family, clients, students, colleagues, and friends for contributions to World Reflexology Foundation, Reflexology Disaster Response Group, Reflexology Research Analysis and Categorization Project, PMS Reflexology Research Study, World Reflexology Week, American Academy of Reflexology; for opening doors across America and internationally; as well as for other endeavors. Ronney Aden, Aetherius, Laura Aho, Denis Alvino, OMD, LAc, William Barry, Nancy Bartlett, Joanna Blanquart-White, Fred Burlson, Tina Bystrom, Cindy Carlin, Joan Cass, Sara Chameides, Lisa Chan LAc, Ginger Clack, Stefanie Cook, Beryl Crane, Alice Daniels, Maryejo Del Meijer, Jan Deutsch, W. Eugen Dietrich, Helga Dittmann, Garnet Dupoit, Randy Ellis, Father Josef Eugster, Yvonne Evans, Adrian Fahey, Virginia Farwell, Peter Frandsen, Ramona French, Linda Friedman, Bill and Kay Jean Furlong, Phyllis Garvey, Bernadette Gessner, Tami Goulet, Jan Grub, Karen Hageman, Lori Hanna, Cathi Harley, Paul Harvey, Lynn Hatswell, David Henry, Lisa Hensell, Tamaki Hori, Nancie Hines, Debbie Hitt, Maureen Holdaway, Cheryl Holyk, Zhang Hongjing, Christine Issel, Jan James, Kelly Jarrell, Janis Jay, Kim Jenner, Dr. Tsuneo Kaneko, Madonna Kauffman, Bonny Kemper, Jane Kerns, Caroline Klem, Dorthe Krogsgaard, Jane Mary Lanverman, Judy and Terry Leavitt, Barel Lottermoser, Phyllisann Maguire, PhD, James Mally, ND, Michele Martin-Cuatt, Mariani Shuilan May, Russell McAllister, Irene Melnyk, Michele Milder, Jeannie Mintin, June Motzer, Teresa Nead, Ahmos Netanel, Laura Norman, Terry Oleson, PhD, Laura Lee Ostrowski, Marie Louise Penchoen, Eliza Pfister, Aloisia Pollock, Michael Rainone, Ron Reeves, Jennifer Reinbrecht, Kathy Reynolds, Ross Riddell, Dick Rigby, Ray Rivera, Sandra Rogers, Paul and Madalena Rudé, Bill Runquist, Stefanie Sabounchian, Claudia Serna, Pam Skeggs, Dawn Smith, Suzann Stahl, Sharon Stathis, Janet Stetser, Jan Styles, Ko Tan, Lee Anthony Taylor, Geraldine Thompson, Jude Unegbu, Kelly Urso, Anneke Van't Wout, Robin Varga, Thijs Versteegh, Mary Von Ranker, Sum Yee Wang, Tom Wilkins, Mitta Wise, Laura Woitte, John Wong, DPM, and Hang Xiongwen. For guidance and support while creating this book, thanks to Marilyn Allen, Jonny Bowden, Todd Clapp, Kevin Marie Fuller, Karyn Gerhard, Elizabeth June Hill, Linzy Kearbey, William Thomas, and Christy Wagner. Thanks to all who came before and all who will follow to advance the remarkable field of reflexology and touch the quality of life for billions more. Anyone I have forgotten to mention, thank you for your contributions and understanding.

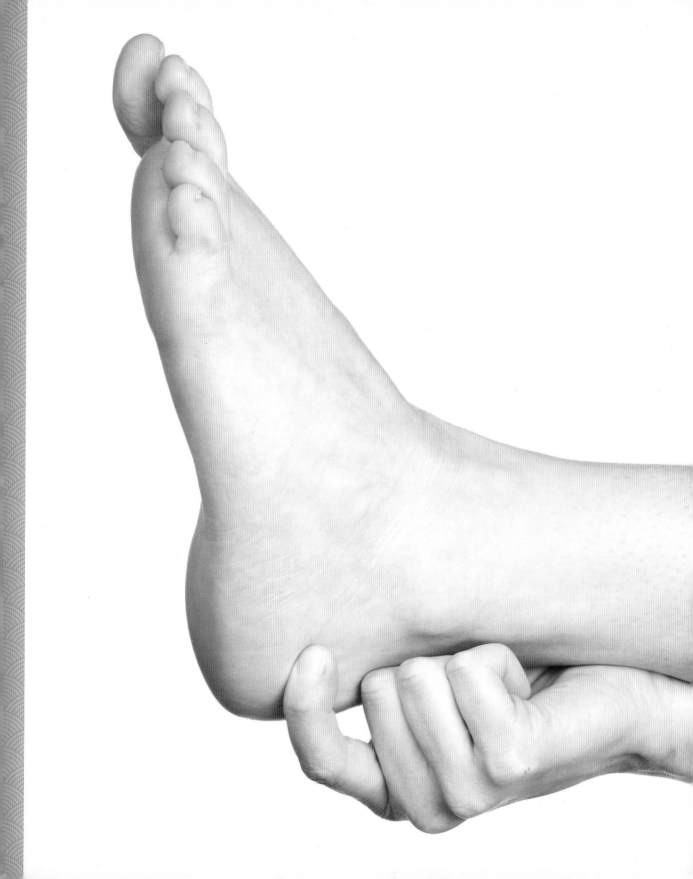

Part 1

Before You Begin

Reflexology, a relatively new field in natural health, is increasingly becoming a highly regarded approach to improved health. Yet there's still so much misinformation about what it is—reflexology is neither massage nor acupressure or acupuncture—and how it works. In Part 1, you learn some fascinating facts about what reflexology really is and the many benefits you can gain from its practice. You also find the answers to some questions you might have about this unique touch therapy as well as some commonsense cautions to be mindful of.

What Is Reflexology?

The human body is a wonderful, amazing thing. It was created with "pressure maps" on the feet, hands, and ears that mimic the shape of the whole body. These maps plot out numerous areas thought to correspond to other parts of the body. Touching and applying pressure to these areas on the feet, hands, and ears can result in health benefits in the related parts of the body.

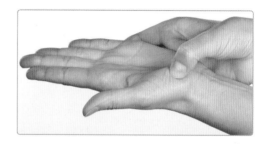

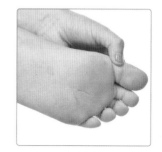

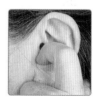

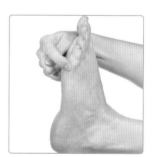

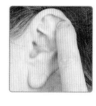

That's the basics of reflexology—applying pressure on specific parts of your feet, hands, and ears to provide relief from pain, discomfort, or other issues throughout the rest of your body. Reflexology can lower stress, enhance relaxation, and provide relief of myriad aliments—all by simply applying pressure to certain areas of your feet, hands, and ears.

Reflexology Terms

Reflexology doesn't have much specialized jargon or unusual words you need to learn and remember, but here are some common terms you'll see used throughout the book:

reflex   A specific location that, when touched, triggers the body to have a response in the related part of the body.

reflex area   A large area on the feet, hands, or ears that corresponds to a large part of the body, such as the shoulders.

reflex point   A small, specific area on the feet, hands, or ears that corresponds to another, small part of the body, such as specific teeth.

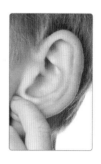

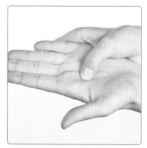

reflexing   The action of applying pressure with your fingers and thumbs (or sometimes special tools) to the feet, hands, or ears.

reflexing technique   One of several ways of using your fingers and thumbs (or sometimes special tools) to apply pressure during a reflexology session.

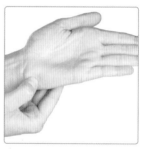

The map of the body wasn't realized until relatively recently, in the twentieth century. In 1917, American William FitzGerald, MD, came up with the vertical zones of the feet and hands. A collaborator of Dr. FitzGerald's, Joe Shelby Riley, MD, came up with horizontal zones of the feet and hands in 1924. These two discoveries formed the foundation of foot and hand reflexology. In 1957, Paul Nogier, MD, of Lyon, France, was the first documented person to suggest the image of the body upside down on the outer ear. Two years later, a research team in Nanjing, China, validated Dr. Nogier's findings and came up with a second, equally valid ear reflex map.

What Reflexology Is—and Is Not

Those unfamiliar with reflexology sometimes confuse it with massage or acupressure. Although both of these are wonderful therapies, reflexology is quite a bit different.

Whereas massage deals mainly with the "superficial tissues"—the blood circulation, lymphatic flow, and musculature of the body—reflexology helps those plus the organs, glands, and structures inside the head, chest, and abdomen. And acupressure, a reflex therapy, identifies long, thin energy lines that run up and down the length of the body, upon which approximately 800 acupressure points lie. Only one of these points, kidney 1, is on the bottom of the feet, and very few on the rest of the feet and hands. None are on the ears.

By contrast, reflexology identifies pressure points on your feet, called *reflexes,* for every part of your body. Another complete reflex map of your body is on your hands, and a third complete map is located on your outer ears.

Working with all three reflexology maps—on your feet, hands, and ears—during the same session provides better results than isolating just one area. And the benefits occur sooner, and last longer, when you work all three areas. For the most effective results, it's best to start with one area (such as the hands); progress to the next area (say, the ears); work the third area (the feet); and return a number of times to the same reflexes in the feet, hands, and ears during the session. You discover more about these different concepts throughout this book.

How Reflexology Works

Theories abound to explain how reflexology works. The main school of thought—based on research—is that reflexology works through the body's nervous system.

Substance P

Your feet, hands, and ears contain reflex areas that correspond to other parts and systems all over and throughout your body. Biopsies have been taken of these areas from the feet of people who have health challenges in the reflex area's corresponding part or system. The results of these biopsies revealed that the reflex area on the foot had a substantially larger number of nerve fibers than that same part of the foot would have in a person without the health issue.

To explain this, one biochemical theory suggests that nerve endings in a reflex related to a health-challenged area of the body produce higher amounts of a chemical called Substance P—the *P* stands for "pain."

Tying together these two ideas, the thinking is that when a health issue occurs someplace in the body, an increased number of nerve endings grow at the related reflex on the feet, hands, and ears, and a larger amount of the neurotransmitter Substance P is produced as well.

A Chain Reaction

When delicate nerve endings in the feet, hands, and ears, are touched in a certain way, messages travel to the central nervous system and into the brain, where they trigger responses in related parts of the body. For example, if you have an upset stomach and you apply pressure to the stomach reflex areas on your feet, hands, and ears, chances are, you'll feel noticeably better.

Part of the reason seems to be that through touch—using just your fingers and thumbs—you help dissipate the accumulated Substance P and other chemicals produced by the extra amount of nerve endings. As you break down the irritating chemicals around the nerve endings, pain and discomfort to the nerve endings is reduced, too.

As a result, the message transmitted through the nerve endings becomes a more soothing and relaxing one. A chain reaction then occurs: your nerves relax, and your muscles relax, which helps your blood vessels relax, meaning more blood can flow. As more blood flows, more oxygen and nutrients are carried to cells throughout your body. As your cells get more oxygen and nutrients, they produce their own chemicals more optimally. Throughout your body, everything just works *better*.

How much pressure should you apply when performing reflexology? That depends. If you or the person upon which you're performing reflexology prefer receiving light pressure, keep it light. If you prefer deeper pressure, that's fine, too. Start with lighter pressure, and as the tissue and muscles closer to the skin begin to soften, you can gradually go deeper, with no more effort or strain on your fingers and thumbs. (More on applying pressure later.)

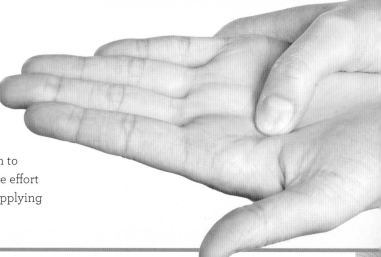

Therapeutic Touch

Although you can use special reflexology tools to help apply pressure in some cases (more on such tools later), most often all you really need to perform reflexology well are your thumbs and fingers.

With just the pads and tips of your thumbs and fingers, you can feel the areas of your feet, hands, and ears where extra nerve endings are located—as well as a buildup of irritating chemicals around the nerve endings. By touching these areas, you can learn exactly where to reflex.

With your touch, you have better control of how much pressure you apply to the tissues of your feet, hands, and ears. Additionally, with your touch, you usually can actually feel the irregular tissues change as you dissipate the underlying irritating chemicals.

The Benefits of Reflexology

The millions of people around the world who have experienced reduced pain, less discomfort, lowered stress levels, and better health and well-being—all thanks to reflexology—can attest to its many benefits. What's more, hundreds of studies performed worldwide have shown, time and time again, the healing results of this touch therapy. Let's take a closer look at what reflexology might be able to do for you.

Stress Reduction

For a moment, think about how busy your life can become with taking care of your house; shopping; cooking; eating; washing dishes; doing laundry; dusting, vacuuming, and cleaning your home; helping your spouse, children, other relatives, neighbors, or friends; staying up late reading, watching TV, or being on the computer; commuting; dealing with daily pressures and stresses at work; handling money and financial issues; taking care of necessary weekend chores; and in general, living a relentless, busy pace, day after day, week after week, month after month, year after year, and decade after decade. Imagine the accumulation of stress throughout every part of your body due to living this way.

Most people who have never experienced reflexology before are amazed at how profoundly relaxing reflexology can be and how it can help plummet their stress levels.

Better Sleep

Next to stress reduction, the most commonly reported benefit of reflexology is better, deeper, and more refreshing sleep. When you sleep better, you feel better, function better, think more clearly, and have a more positive attitude and better disposition throughout your day.

Improved Circulation

As you experience stress reduction and better sleep, a natural consequence is improved circulation because, as muscles relax, blood vessels also relax, permitting more oxygen and nutrients to go to the estimated 75 trillion cells in your body.

Detoxification

As every cell of your body metabolizes oxygen and a broad range of nutrients, they also release toxins. With improved circulation, more toxins are released from the cells and removed from your body. With fewer toxins, you naturally feel better.

Improved Organ and Gland Function

As your circulation improves, more oxygen and nutrients get into every cell of your body, toxins are taken away, and organs and glands have a better chance to function and produce their chemistry. For example, your brain produces more of its feel-good chemicals, your digestive tract produces more digestive juices, your adrenal glands produce more adrenaline, your pancreas produces more insulin, and so on throughout your body.

Many people use reflexology as a mini feel-good stress-reduction break each week. You can, too!

Pain Reduction and Elimination

As tension is reduced and your body does a better job of producing its wide range of chemicals, pain is often reduced or eliminated, too.

Studies have documented pain reduction in areas such as your abdomen, ankles, elbows, hands, head, hips, knees, legs, neck, sciatic nerve, shoulders, and teeth and gums, plus conditions such as allergies, arthritis, asthma, cancer, colitis, gallstones, menstrual cramps, premenstrual syndrome, and urinary issues—to mention just a few.

Increased Range of Motion

Another natural consequence of stress reduction and profound relaxation is increased range of motion. Don't be surprised if, after several reflexology sessions, you're better able to turn your neck; raise your arms; and experience more movement in your legs, hips, and spine.

Normalization of Body Functions

You might have noticed that sometimes when you get stressed, you feel more hyper, anxious, or nervous. At other times, you might feel more sluggish, sleepy, and slower than usual.

Reflexology tends to normalize your body functions. This means that if stresses cause your body to become hyperactive, reflexology tends to help it slow down to normal. If you feel you've become sluggish, reflexology can help bring you back up to normal.

Improved Wellness

By reducing the accumulated stress in your body; with better sleep, improved circulation, and detoxification; and with your cells, organs, and glands doing their jobs better, your natural immunity and defenses should be stronger, helping prevent aches, pains, flus, colds, and other health issues so you're healthier and have a better allover wellness.

Reflexology can help with all of this. With reflexology, you can feel good, be more productive, have a higher quality of life, and be better equipped to deal with all aspects of your life.

Warnings and Cautions

Whenever you perform reflexology—on yourself or on someone else—you want to be careful to maintain good hygiene when skin touches skin. More importantly, you want to be sure to notice anything on or under the skin, or any condition elsewhere in the body, that might require a lighter or different touch—or indicate you maybe shouldn't perform reflexology right now at all.

In this section, you discover when it's best to use a lighter touch when performing reflexology, and when you should wait until a condition has healed, lessened, or changed before attempting to touch.

Cuts, Lacerations, Abrasions, and Bruises

Avoid touching broken skin, such as cuts, lacerations, and abrasions. Performing reflexology on these areas can aggravate, infect, make more painful, or interfere with the body's self-healing process. Also avoid working on bruised areas for the same reasons.

Skin Infections

Stay away from any part of the feet, hands, or ears that might have an infection—or even *look* like they might have an infection. You don't want to risk spreading the infection to other parts of the body, if you're working on someone else, or catching it yourself.

Skin Conditions

Avoid working on areas that might be affected with certain skin conditions. On the feet, hands, and (much less often) the outer ears, do not perform reflexology on areas that might have rashes, psoriasis, or eczema. It's unlikely that you'll spread these conditions, or catch them yourself, but you could cause additional discomfort by touching.

Strained and Sprains

A sprain is an overly stretched or torn ligament; a strain is an overly stretched or torn muscle or tendon. Either can occur in the feet or hands. Touching a strain or sprained area can hurt more and aggravate the situation.

> When working on arthritic parts of the body, always reflex *lightly,* if at all.

Injured Bones and Joints

Touching bruised or broken bones or painful joints, such as those in people with arthritis in their feet or hands, can slow the healing process. Sometimes it even can interfere with it to the point of making the condition worse.

Irritated Nerves

If touched incorrectly, neuroma, or a pinched nerve, between the long bones of the feet, and conditions such as carpal tunnel syndrome in and around the wrists can hurt and be made worse. Take a light touch around these areas.

Varicose Veins

Touching varicose veins can cause more pain and make the condition worse by breaking more of the delicate little one-way values inside the veins.

After Foot, Hand, or Ear Surgery

Don't work on parts of the feet, hands, or ears that have had surgery recently. Even though the skin that was cut during surgery might have healed and look just fine, the muscles, ligaments, tendons, bones, joints, nerves, and blood and lymphatic vessels below the skin might not yet be fully healed. Working on such areas can hurt and even make the condition worse.

Advanced Type II Diabetes

People with diabetes can have a variety of situations develop in their feet, including poor circulation, nerve damage, neuropathy, peeling or cracking skin, calluses, sores, ulcers, and in the extreme, amputation.

Many reflexologists, including me, have worked on diabetics successfully. However, before doing so, it's wise to ask if any of these conditions are present. When in doubt, check with a health-care provider. Or opt for hand and ear reflexology only, and skip the feet.

Hemophilia

It's best to get a doctor's authorization before working on people with hemophilia. And even after you do, reflex quite lightly until you find out how the person responds.

It's best not to work directly on such areas for at least a year after surgery. If in doubt, get permission from the attending physician.

Warnings and Cautions *(continued)*

Alternating High/Low Blood Pressure

If someone with this rare condition is going into a low blood pressure phase, the extra relaxation reflexology provides could cause him or her to pass out. Before reflexing someone with alternating high and low blood pressure, be sure they get their doctor's authorization.

Lymphatic Cancer

There's a discussion among reflexologists today on the wisdom of performing reflexology on someone with lymphatic cancer. One school of thought suggests that relaxing the body with reflexology helps lymphatic fluids flow through the lymphatic vessels more, potentially carrying with it more cancer cells. The other school claims that lymphatic fluids are flowing through the body anyway, and reflexology can help the body distress, relax, and better produce its white blood cells and other beneficial chemicals.

If in doubt, talk to a doctor. If the doctor doesn't know about reflexology, you can explain that reflexology provides profound relaxation throughout the body.

During the First Trimester of Pregnancy

Reflexology can be relaxing and help with morning sickness and other issues that come up during pregnancy, but use caution during the first trimester. During this sometimes-delicate time, you don't want to aggravate or cause any potential problems for mother or baby.

Therefore, it's commonly agreed upon in the reflexology community to either avoid working on the uterine reflexes on the feet, hands, and ears during the first trimester of pregnancy or to do so quite lightly and for short periods of time.

The Importance of Drinking Water

As you apply pressure to the feet, hands, and ears, toxins can be released from the cells in these areas as well as throughout the body. Drinking plenty of fluids, especially water, helps your body flush out the released toxins Increase your fluids the day you reflex and for a few days after if you feel you need it. People who do prolonged reflexology on themselves and don't drink plenty of fluids sometimes can feel little bit off later in the day or the next day.

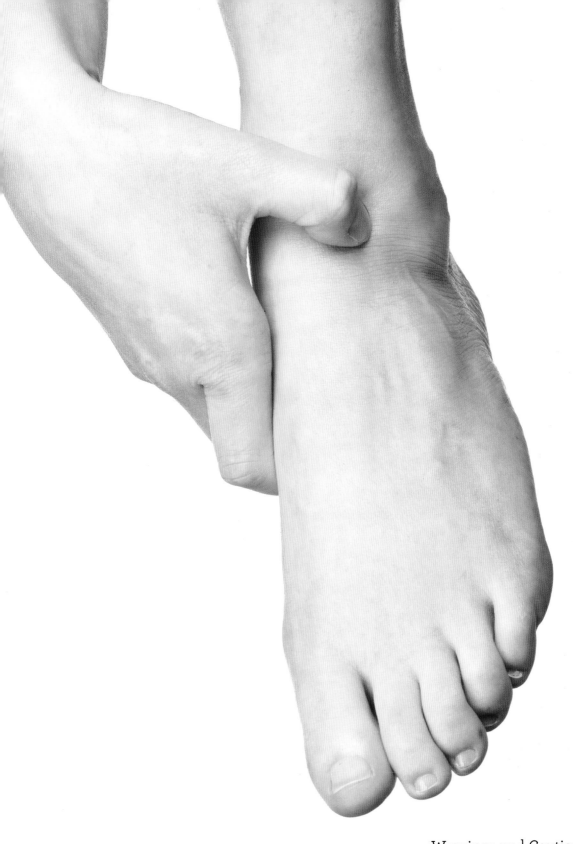

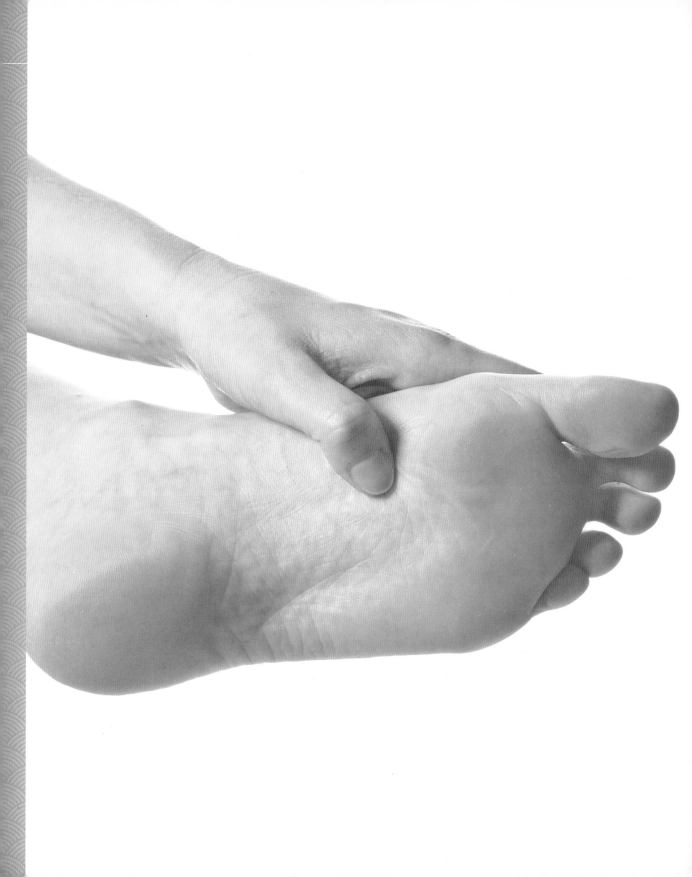

Part 2

Reflexology Basics

At its core, reflexology is about touching and applying pressure to certain parts of your feet, hands, and ears to provide relief of pain or discomfort in other parts of your body or to boost the health of those corresponding areas. But how do you know which spots on your feet, hands, and ears align with which other areas in your body? That's where reflexology maps come in. These detailed illustrations show where all the various reflexes are on your feet, hands, and ears. And when you don't have a map handy, you can still know in general where to reflex for what ails you by thinking of your body as divided into specific regions and understanding where those regions align with your feet, hands, and ears.

The Foot Maps

The reflexes on your right foot correspond to the right half of your body. Reflexing the tips of your toes helps the top of your head, and working on the rest of your toes helps the right half of your head and neck. Reflexing the big knuckles at the base of your toes aids your shoulders, lungs, and chest muscles. Working on your arch helps your upper abdomen. Your heel holds reflexes for the lower part of your abdomen and torso, and the outer edge of your foot corresponds to your right arm and leg. The inner edge of your foot aligns with your spinal column.

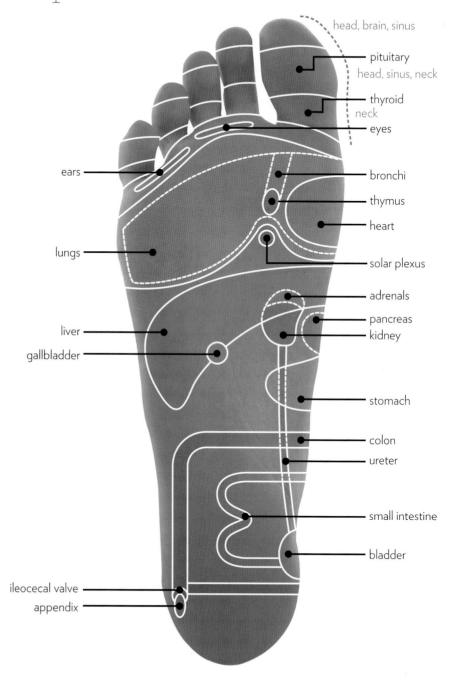

head, brain, sinus

pituitary
head, sinus, neck

thyroid
neck

eyes

ears

bronchi

thymus

heart

lungs

solar plexus

adrenals

pancreas

kidney

liver

gallbladder

stomach

colon

ureter

small intestine

bladder

ileocecal valve

appendix

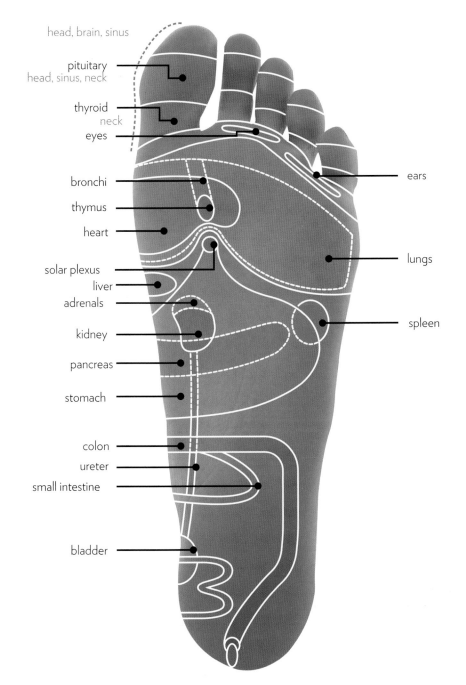

head, brain, sinus

pituitary
head, sinus, neck

thyroid
neck

eyes

bronchi

thymus

heart

solar plexus

liver

adrenals

kidney

pancreas

stomach

colon

ureter

small intestine

bladder

ears

lungs

spleen

The reflexes on your left foot align with the left half of your body. Reflexes on the tips of your toes correspond with the top of your head, your toes align with your head and neck, and the big knuckles where your toes join your foot hold reflexes for your chest. Your arch is home to reflexes for your upper abdomen. Reflexing your heel helps the lower part of your abdomen and torso. The outer edge of your foot aligns with your left arm and leg, and reflexing the inner edge of your foot, from your big toe to your heel, benefits your spine.

The Foot Maps *(continued)*

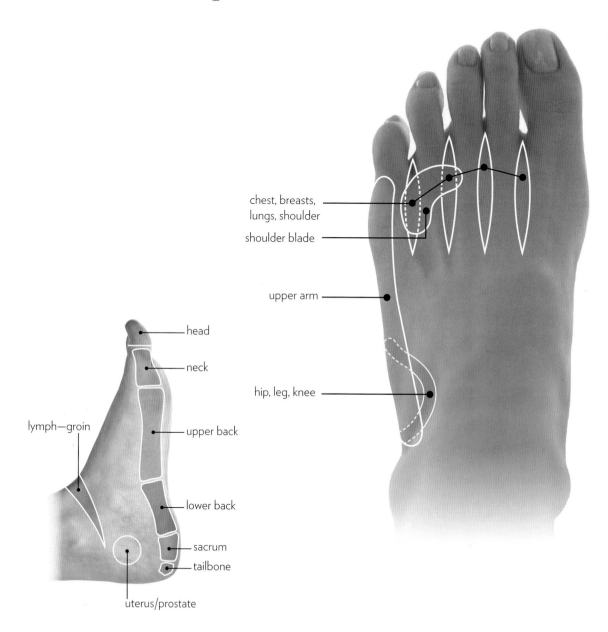

chest, breasts, lungs, shoulder

shoulder blade

upper arm

hip, leg, knee

head

neck

lymph—groin

upper back

lower back

sacrum

tailbone

uterus/prostate

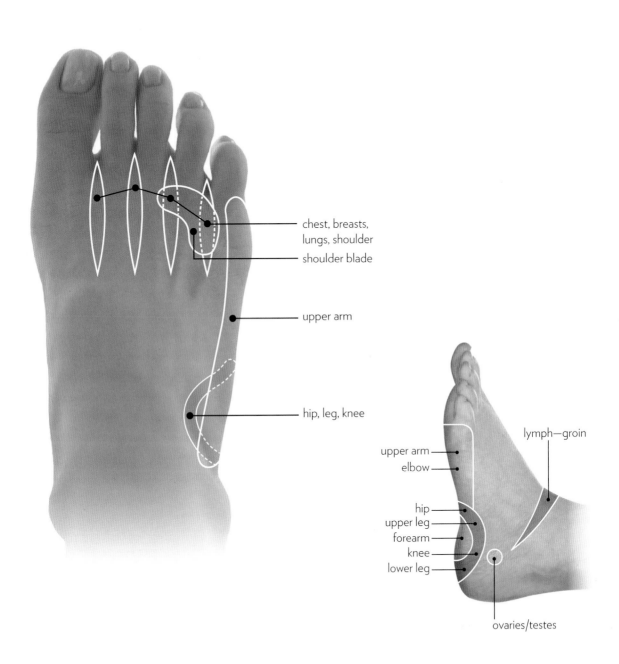

chest, breasts,
lungs, shoulder

shoulder blade

upper arm

hip, leg, knee

upper arm

elbow

lymph—groin

hip

upper leg

forearm

knee

lower leg

ovaries/testes

The Hand Maps

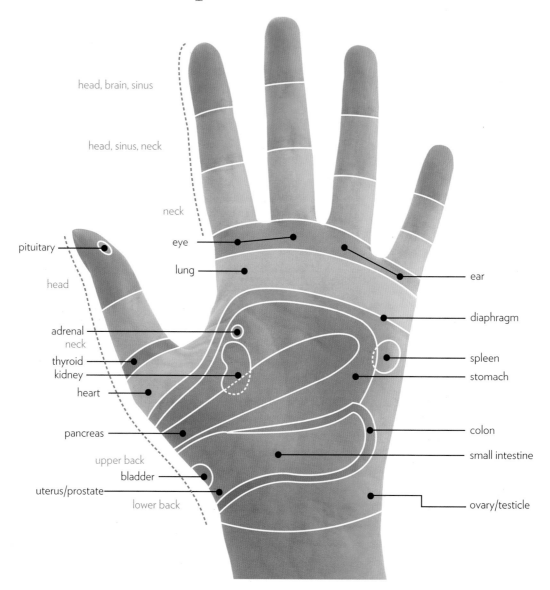

head, brain, sinus

head, sinus, neck

neck

pituitary

eye

head

lung

ear

adrenal

neck

diaphragm

thyroid

spleen

kidney

stomach

heart

pancreas

colon

upper back

small intestine

bladder

uterus/prostate

lower back

ovary/testicle

Working reflexes on your left hand benefits the left half of your body. The reflexes on the tips of your fingers align with the top of your head, your fingers match up with your head and neck, and the big knuckles where your fingers join your hand hold reflexes for your chest. Your palm corresponds to your upper abdomen, and the heel of your hand is home to reflexes for the lower part of your abdomen and torso. The outer edge of your hand carries reflexes for your left arm and leg, and the inner edge contains reflexes for your spine.

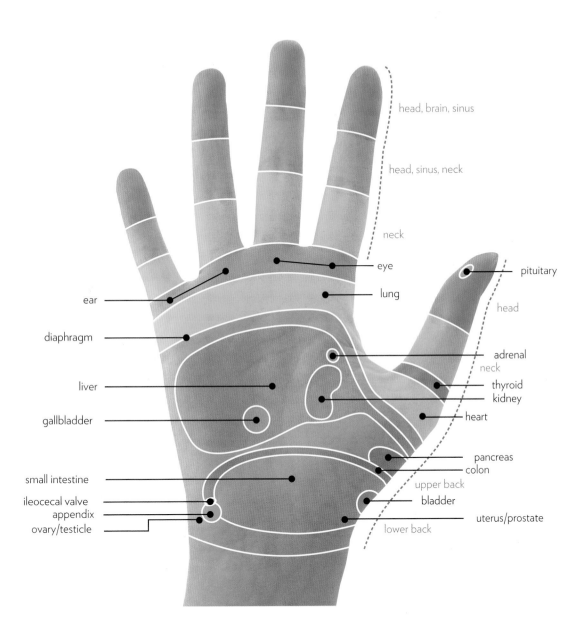

head, brain, sinus

head, sinus, neck

neck

eye

lung

pituitary

ear

head

diaphragm

adrenal

neck

liver

thyroid

kidney

gallbladder

heart

pancreas

colon

upper back

small intestine

ileocecal valve

bladder

appendix

ovary/testicle

uterus/prostate

lower back

The reflexes on your right hand correspond to the right half of your body. Reflexing the tips of your fingers helps the top of your head, and the rest of your fingers and thumb hold reflexes for the right half of your head and neck. Working on your big knuckles helps your shoulders, lungs, and chest muscles. Your palm aligns with your upper abdomen, and the heel of your hand contains reflexes for your lower abdomen and torso. The outer edge of your right hand aligns with your right arm and leg, and the inner edge benefits your spine.

The Hand Maps (continued)

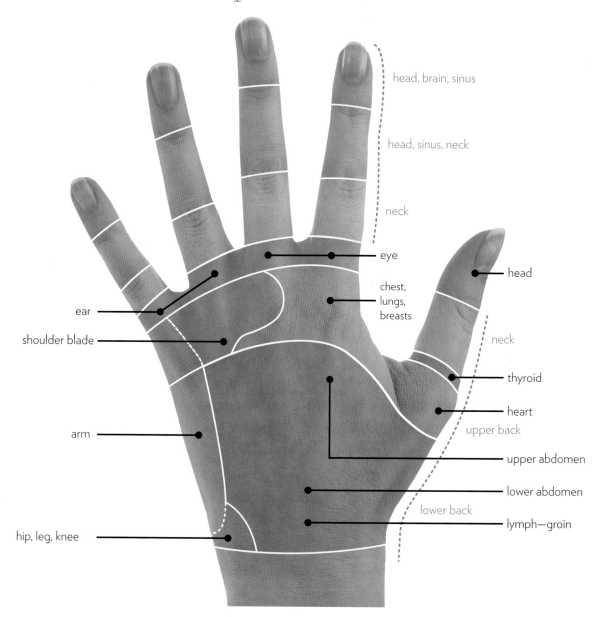

head, brain, sinus

head, sinus, neck

neck

eye

chest, lungs, breasts

head

ear

shoulder blade

neck

thyroid

heart

upper back

arm

upper abdomen

lower abdomen

lower back

lymph—groin

hip, leg, knee

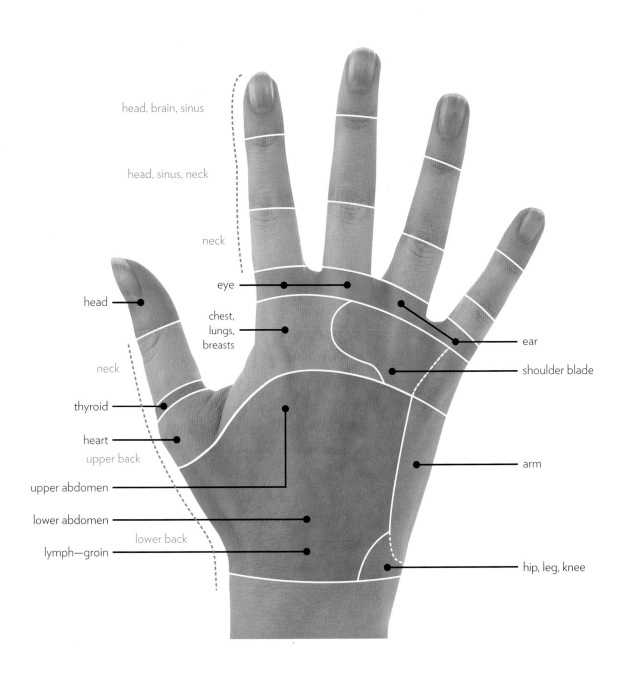

head, brain, sinus

head, sinus, neck

neck

eye

head

chest,
lungs,
breasts

neck

thyroid

heart

upper back

upper abdomen

lower abdomen

lower back

lymph—groin

ear

shoulder blade

arm

hip, leg, knee

The Ear Map

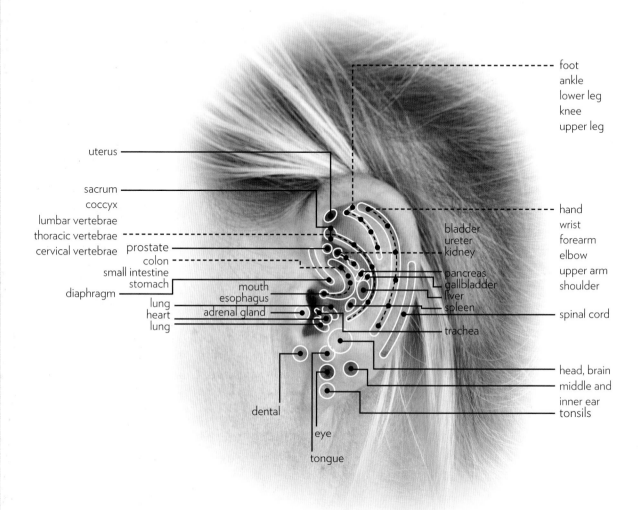

uterus

sacrum
coccyx
lumbar vertebrae
thoracic vertebrae
cervical vertebrae — prostate
colon
small intestine
stomach
diaphragm
lung
heart
lung

mouth
esophagus
adrenal gland

dental

eye

tongue

foot
ankle
lower leg
knee
upper leg

hand
wrist
forearm
elbow
upper arm
shoulder

bladder
ureter
kidney

pancreas
gallbladder
liver
spleen

spinal cord

trachea

head, brain
middle and
inner ear
tonsils

From the bottom of your ear to the top, the areas on your ears correspond to areas throughout your body, just like with the foot and hand maps. Your earlobe contains reflexes for your head and brain. The middle part of your ear holds reflexes for the middle part of your body. Moving up your ear you'll find reflexes for your lower back, and near the top of your ear are reflexes for your feet and toes.

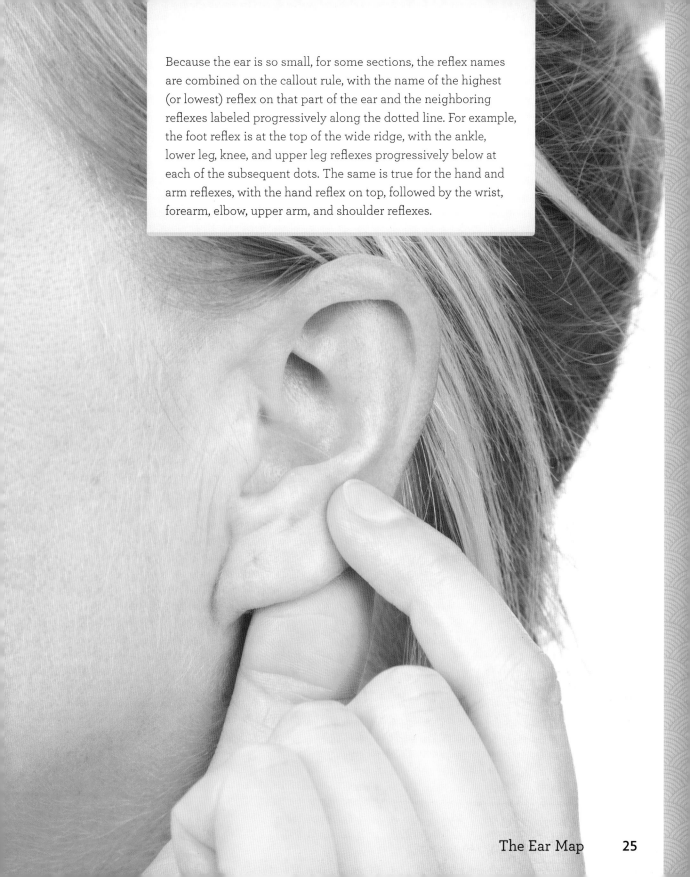

Because the ear is so small, for some sections, the reflex names are combined on the callout rule, with the name of the highest (or lowest) reflex on that part of the ear and the neighboring reflexes labeled progressively along the dotted line. For example, the foot reflex is at the top of the wide ridge, with the ankle, lower leg, knee, and upper leg reflexes progressively below at each of the subsequent dots. The same is true for the hand and arm reflexes, with the hand reflex on top, followed by the wrist, forearm, elbow, upper arm, and shoulder reflexes.

The Seven Regions of the Body

When it comes to reflexology, you can imagine your body divided into seven main regions: head and neck, chest, upper abdomen, lower abdomen/pelvic area, arms, legs, and spine. When you have a health issue in one of these regions, you can work on each of your body's anatomical systems by reflexing for that system, such as your entire lymphatic system. Or you can focus on one specific part of that system, such as the lymph nodes in your neck. You also could work by specific issue, such as focusing on the reflexes for your appendix on your feet, hands, and ears.

If something in your leg hurts, for example, you can work on the leg reflex region on your feet, hands, and ears. This way you don't need to know exactly where the knee, lower leg, or ankle reflexes are (although that's helpful information to learn). Plus, if your knee is hurting, the upper and lower parts of your leg are likely being stressed as well. By reflexing the broad area, you reflex for everything affected.

The Head and Neck Region

For your head and neck, work on each of your toes, especially your big toes; each of your fingers, especially your thumbs; your earlobes; and the lower 1 inch (2.5cm) of your ear's middle ridge. This benefits your brain, which affects everything in your body, and your pituitary gland, which impacts your body's other endocrine glands. The nerves that begin at the base of your brain, the 12 cranial nerves, impact the head and neck as well. Your eyes, nasal passages, middle and inner ears, pineal and pituitary glands, sinuses, tonsils, tongue, teeth and gums, thyroid and parathyroid glands, and throat, among others, are also included. Externally, your jaw, nose, and outer ears also benefit.

The Chest Region

For your chest, work the ball and pad of your feet and the grooves on top of your feet. On your hands, work the palm side of your big knuckles where your fingers join your hand plus the grooves on the back of your hand. On your ears, work your lower valley, and halfway up your middle ridge. This benefits your heart, lungs, trachea, esophagus, and thymus. Your external chest also benefits: your breasts, pectoral muscles, ribs, and collar bones, plus everything behind your chest—your upper back muscles, shoulders, shoulder blades, etc.

The Upper Abdominal Region

For your upper abdomen, work on the arch of your feet and the soft part of the palm of your hands. On your ears, work your inner ridge, the root of your outer ridge, and part of your upper valley for your inner abdomen, and for the musculature of your outer abdomen, work midway up your middle ridge, slightly above the external chest reflexes. This benefits your diaphragm, stomach, pancreas, spleen, kidneys, liver, gallbladder, and more. Externally this works your abdominal muscles and lower ribs.

Inside many of the bones in your body is a softer center called marrow, where most of your blood is made. Even if you don't have any health issues in your arms, legs, or spine, reflex these areas so they're optimally equipped to produce marrow and blood and boost your body's overall health.

The Lower Abdominal Region

For everything in your lower abdominal area, work your heels, including the sides, the heel of your hands, and the outer and inner edge of your hands near your wrist. On your ears, reflex your upper valley and triangular valley for your internal abdomen, and for your external abdomen, work your upper middle ridge and narrow ridge. This benefits most of your small intestines, ileocecal valve, appendix, colon (large intestine), rectum, most of your urinary system, and your reproductive system internally. Externally, it helps your hips, hip bones, pelvic bones, lower abdominal muscles, and gluteal muscles (buttocks), to name a few.

The Arm Region

For your arms, reflex the outer edge of your feet, from just below your small toes to your heels. On your hands, work on the outer edge, from just below the base of your little fingers almost to your wrists. On your ears, reflex your outer valley, from above the base all the way up to the top. This benefits the skin, muscles, bones, nerves, and blood vessels in your arms plus the lymphatic vessels and lymph nodes in your elbow. In addition, your upper arms, elbows, forearms, wrists, hands, fingers, and thumbs benefit.

The Leg Region

For your legs, reflex below your ankle bone on your feet all the way down to the bottom of your foot. On your hands, reflex the outer edge near your wrist. On your ears, work your wide ridge. This benefits the muscles, bones, nerves, and blood vessels of your upper legs, knees, lower legs, ankles, feet, and toes, plus your lymphatic vessels and lymph nodes behind your knee.

The Spinal Region

For your spinal column, work the inner edge of your feet from your big toes down to your heels. On your hands, focus on the inside edge, from your thumbs down to your wrists. On your ears, reflex the arch of your middle ridge and all of your narrow ridge. This benefits your spinal column, which is made of a series of bones, called vertebrae, and softer discs between each of these bones. Your spinal cord benefits as well as two sets of muscles running along each side of your spinal column.

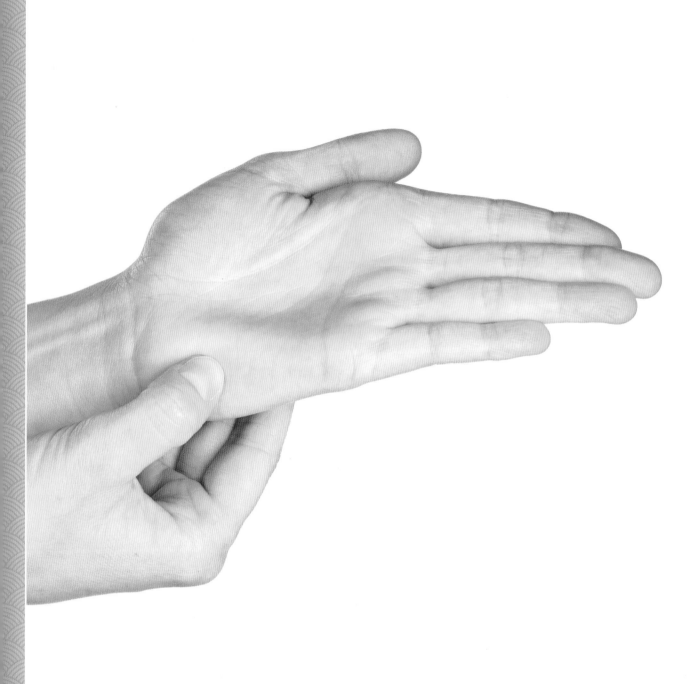

Part 3

Reflexology Techniques

You don't need any special tools or equipment to practice reflexology. (Although you are welcome to use some simple tools for additional benefits, if you like.) All you really need are your feet, hands, and ears to work on and your hands to apply healing touch. However, it does help to know the best setup for your reflexology session, and it's important that you know the proper touch technique so you get the most beneficial results. In this part, you learn the best ways to perform reflexology on the feet, hands, and ears.

Getting into Position

One of the many wonderful things about reflexology is that you can do reflexology work on yourself as well as on someone else.

Reflexology on Yourself

When practicing reflexology on yourself, especially if you're just working for fairly short periods of time, you can be in almost any position you want—standing, sitting, lying down, reclining in an easy chair, in bed, etc.

The most common way of working on your feet would be for you to be in a sitting position, preferably in a chair with no arms, so you can put your foot up on your knee and have plenty of room to move your arms around freely, without interference from the arms of a chair. Let your foot extend past your knee a bit so you easily can reach all areas of your foot and ankle.

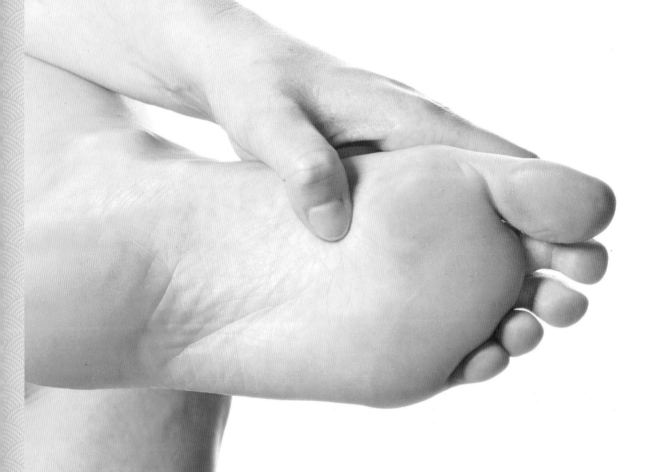

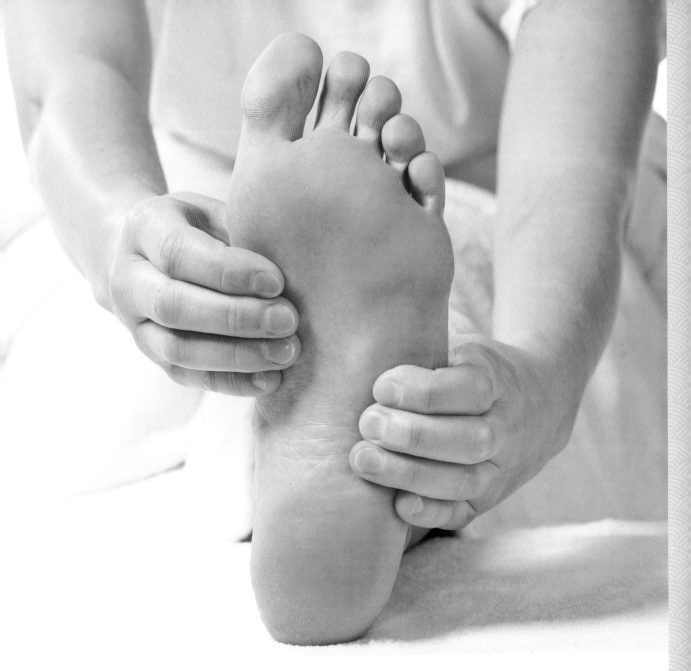

If you're more flexible, or if it would be more comfortable for your knees, you instead could sit on a bed or on the floor with one leg straight out in front of you. Then you could bend at your waist and hips to reach your foot for reflexology work.

Although most of the focus of this book is on teaching you self-help reflexology, or reflexing your own feet, hands, and ears, you easily can adapt any of the instructions throughout to give the gift of reflexology to someone else.

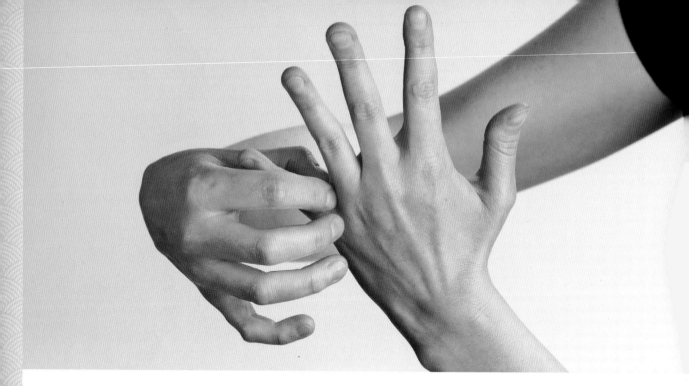

Getting into Position *(continued)*

To work on your hands, you have a few more options. You could work with your hands in front of you, in your lap, or on top of a pillow placed on your lap so your hands are a little higher. If you're sitting at your desk or a table, you can rest your hands on the desk- or tabletop.

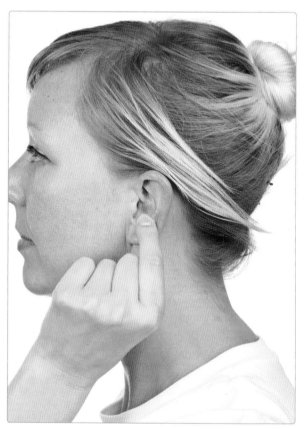

When working on your ears, you can just reach up to work on them, especially if you're only working for short periods of time. However, if you're going to work for more than a few minutes, rest your elbows on a desk- or tabletop so you don't tire your arms and shoulders. Then you can hold reflex points and areas as long as you would like—5, 10, 20, or even 30 minutes at a time—without straining your arms and shoulders.

Reflexology on Someone Else

When you're performing reflexology on someone else, he or she can be positioned in a number of ways—on the floor, in a chair or a recliner (preferably one with no or low arms), or on a bed. Really, once you get comfortable and confident performing reflexology on others, you can adapt to whatever position the recipient is in.

If you're reflexing someone else's feet, and they're sitting in a chair, sit in another chair facing them. Place a third chair between the two of you, and place a pillow or cushion on that chair. Place the recipient's lower legs on the pillow to raise their feet so it's comfortable for you to work on them with your back straight, so you don't have to strain or stoop forward.

If he or she is in a recliner, have them lean back in the chair so their feet come up high enough for you to work on them comfortably. Sit in another chair, positioned at their feet, facing them with your back straight.

For hand reflexology work, move your chair beside the person so you're beside but facing them. Put a pillow on the recipient's lap and work on his or her hands on top of the pillow. You also could work with his or her arm or elbow on the pillow, especially if he or she is in a recliner.

Reflexing someone else's ears when they're seated in a chair is pretty simple. Just stand behind them so you can work on both of their ears at the same time. If the person is in a recliner, you might want to take a seat in a chair behind his or her head so you don't have to stoop low to reflex their ears.

If your recipient is limited to his or her bed, you can still give them a relaxing, healing reflexology session. When reflexing the feet, simply stand or sit at the foot of the bed and work on their feet, keeping your back straight. If necessary, you can put a pillow under their lower legs to raise them high enough to make it comfortable for you to work. For hand reflexology, move your chair next to the edge of the bed so you're beside but facing the recipient. Hold their hand closest to you in one of your own, and reflex with your other hand. To work on his or her other hand, move your chair to his or her other side rather than lean over them. Similar to working on the hands, reflex the recipient's ear one side at a time before moving to the other side.

Techniques for Feet and Hands

The specific moves you use to touch the feet, hands, and ears during reflexology are called *reflexing techniques*. Many different types of techniques are used all over the world. The rolling techniques for foot and hand reflexology explored in this section are ones that have emerged from my reflexology work over the last 30+ years.

The Pitfalls of "Inchworm" Techniques

The most common reflexology technique goes by names such as "inchworm," "thumb walk," "caterpillar," etc. The idea is that you push into a reflex point (often with your thumb), release the pressure, move your thumb forward, and repeat. It's a valid technique and has helped millions of people reap the benefits of reflexology.

One pitfall of this type of technique, however, is that when you release the pressure and move your thumb forward, you skip over a small area that's then left unworked. No matter what technique you use, it's best to go over the same tissue repeatedly. But with the inchworm-type techniques, in order to do a more complete job of getting all the tissue, you have to spend much more time repeatedly going over each part of the feet and hands to ensure you cover all those small spots you skipped over. Because these techniques take so much repetition—and so much time—you can see why most people can only do a single foot reflexology session or a hand reflexology session at one sitting. (The inchworm techniques do not apply to the ears.)

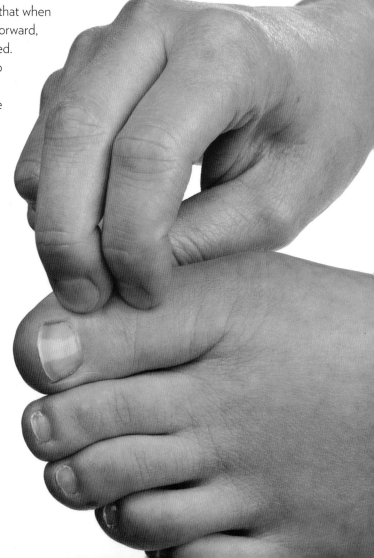

One of my graduates gave me this image, which makes it easier to visualize the idea of a thumb roll: think of a child on a rocking horse. As that child becomes a little older, she learns that as she rolls back on the rocking horse, she can simultaneously scoot the rocking horse forward slightly. By repeating the process, she can move forward some distance. You can do the same thing with the rolling techniques on the feet and hands.

The Benefits of Rolling Techniques

On the other hand (or foot), the rolling techniques I recommend with titles such as "thumb roll," "index finger roll," "index and middle finger roll," and "three finger roll," go over *all* the tissues of your feet and hands, without skipping any spots. This means you don't have to go back over the same tissue as many times, and you can cover much more of the feet and hands more effectively and in a shorter time period. You might even have time to work on your ears, too!

Experienced reflexologists who work on only the feet or only the hands are quite surprised and perplexed to learn that it's not only possible, but also highly effective to work on all three—the feet, hands, and ears—during the same hour-long reflexology session. The main reason this is possible is because of the rolling techniques.

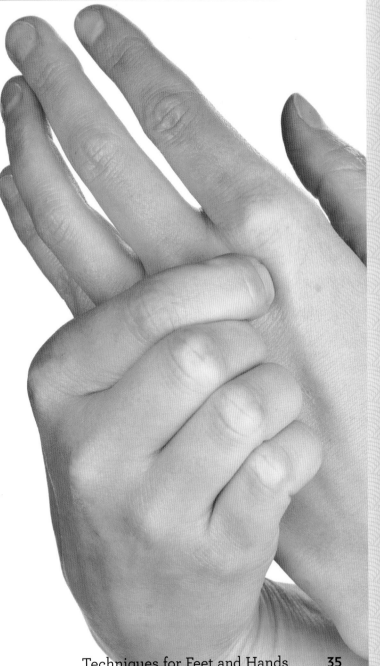

Thumb Roll

The thumb roll is one of the principle techniques you'll use during reflexology. It's one you can use on yourself and on others.

The versatile thumb roll gives you a way to apply pressure on large, soft surfaces, such as the arch of your foot and the palm of your hand, as well as on small, hard surfaces, such as on the knuckles of your toes and fingers.

Use the pad of your thumb to apply pressure to larger areas. Use the tip and corners of your thumb to zero in on smaller, more detailed areas.

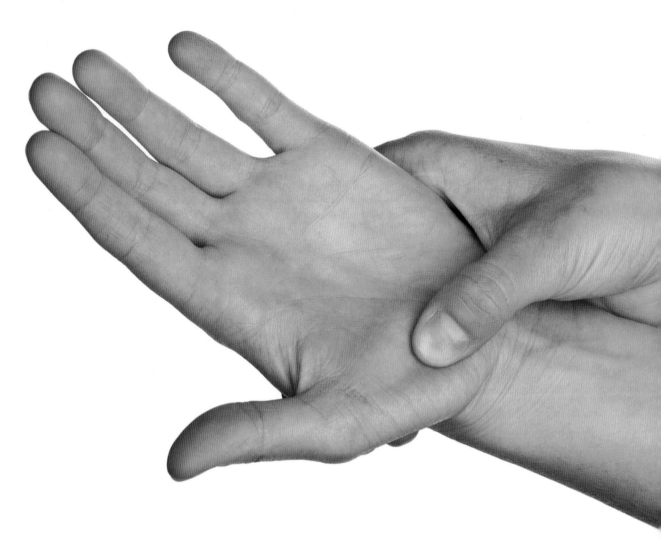

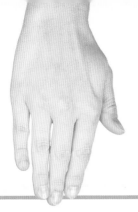
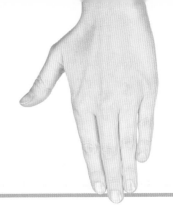

The shorter your thumb and fingernails, the more options you have to work different surfaces of the feet, hands, and ears. In addition, the shorter they are, the less likely you are to cause pain or discomfort to yourself or the person you're working on. Keep your fingernails short to provide a more pleasant experience.

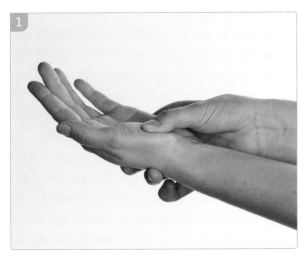

With the pad of your thumb, gently apply pressure.

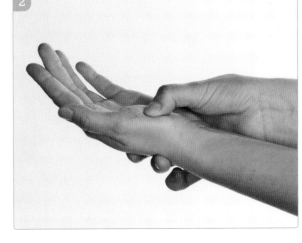

Maintaining the same pressure (not pushing into the tissue harder), roll your thumb, moving the knuckle closet to your thumbnail forward and up partway.

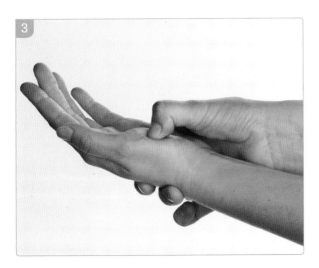

Still maintaining pressure, continue to roll your thumb, moving that same knuckle forward and up, until your thumbnail is straight up and down.

Thumb Roll   37

Index Finger Roll
and Sideways Index Finger Roll

The area around the tip of your index finger, including the sides, can help you do some detailed reflexology work, especially on hard, bony areas of your feet and hands.

Because the size of your index fingertip is so small in comparison to the tip of your thumb, you can use it more effectively to get into small areas, such as between the knuckles at the base of your fingers and toes, as well as in the grooves between the long bones on the tops of your feet and on the backs of your hands.

For the sideways index finger roll, follow the steps for index finger roll but instead of rolling forward, roll from one corner of your fingertip over the edge of your fingertip, to the other corner of your fingertip.

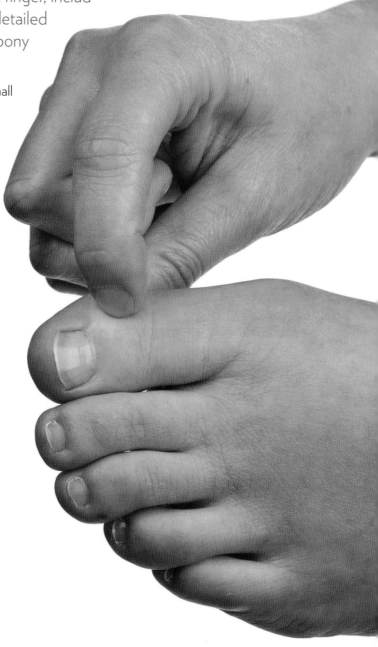

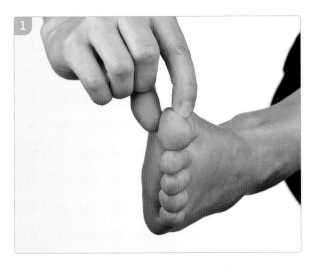

1

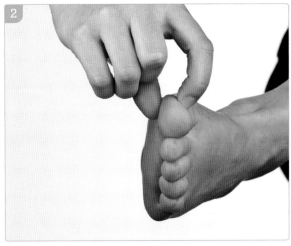

2

Using the part of the pad of your index finger near the tip, gently apply pressure.

Maintaining the same pressure, roll your finger, moving the knuckle closet to your nail forward and partway up.

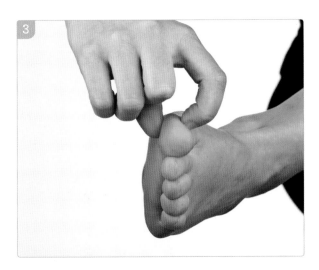

3

Still maintaining pressure, continue to roll your finger, moving your knuckle forward and up, until your fingernail is straight up and down.

The shorter the nails on your index and middle fingers, the more you can work with the bony tips and corners of your fingers and get into the small grooves and spaces on your feet and hands.

Index and Middle Finger Roll

When used together as one unit, your index and middle fingers are stronger than if you use one finger alone.

Your index and middle fingers will never be as strong as your thumb, but they can help you work on some hard, bony surfaces, such as the back of your fingers and tops of your toes. They can also help you reach some areas that might be hard to get to, especially on your feet.

Remember, the shorter the nails on your index and middle fingers, the more you can work with the bony tips and corners of your fingers—and the more you can do more detail work.

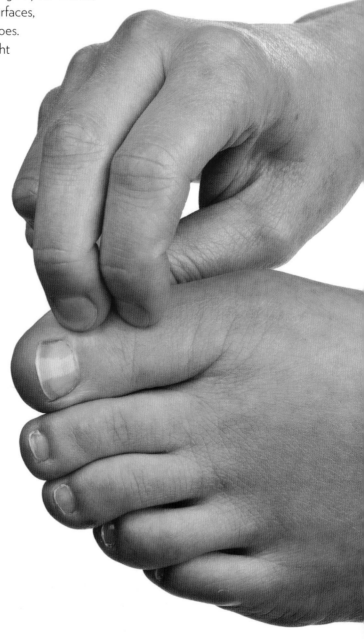

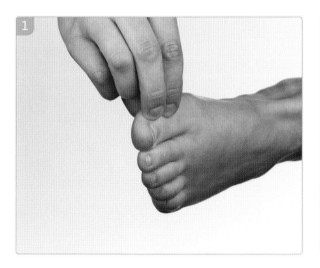

Using the part of the pad near the tips of your index and middle fingers, gently apply pressure.

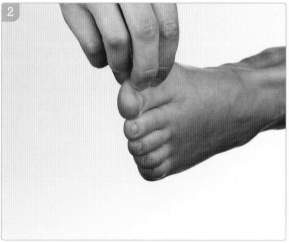

Maintaining the same pressure, roll your fingers, moving the knuckles closet to your fingernails forward and partway up.

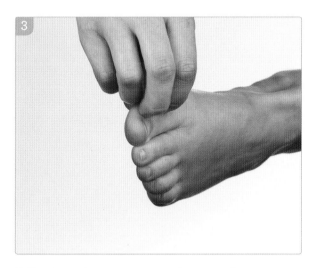

Still maintaining pressure, continue to roll your fingers, moving your knuckles forward and up until your fingernails are straight up and down.

Index and Middle Finger Roll   **41**

Three-Finger Roll

Similar to the index and middle finger roll, this multiple-finger reflexing technique combines the strength in three of your fingers—your index finger, your middle finger, and your ring finger—to allow you to use more targeted pressure when reflexing.

The strong combination of your index, middle, and fingers can help you work on some hard, bony surfaces, such as on the bones that form the grooves on tops of your feet and backs of your hands.

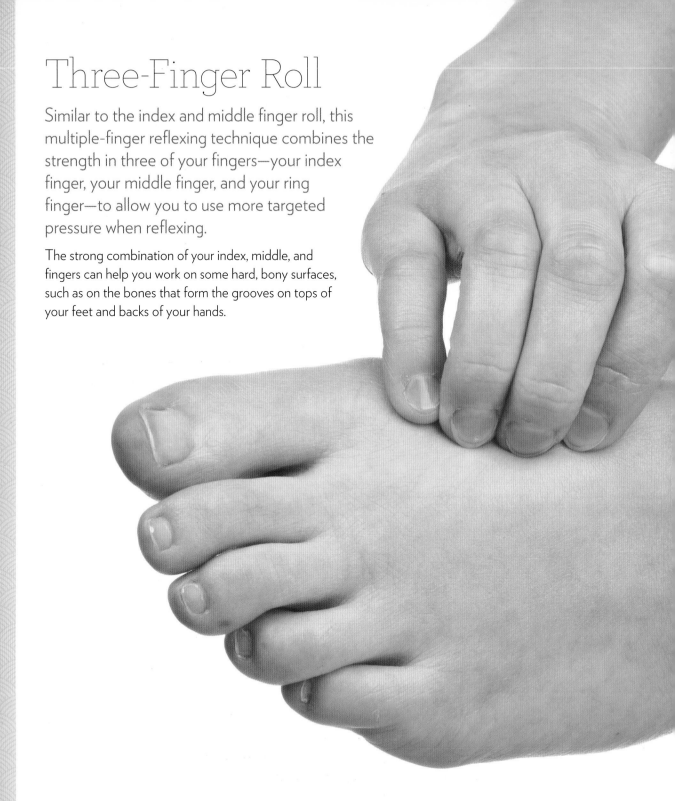

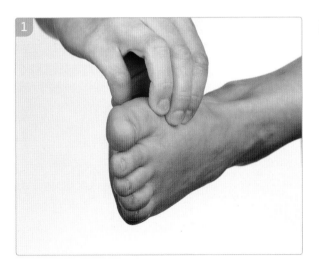

Using the part of the pad near the tips of your index, middle, and ring fingers, apply gentle pressure.

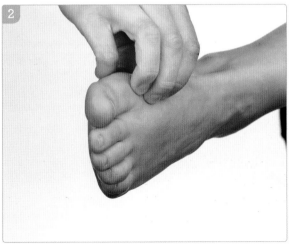

Maintaining the same pressure, roll your fingers as one unit, moving the knuckles closest to your fingernails forward and up partway.

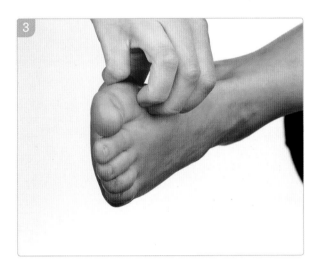

Still maintaining pressure, continue to roll your fingers as a unit, moving your knuckles forward and up until your fingernails are straight up and down.

Three-Finger Roll   **43**

Rotating

This circling technique can be used on the feet, hands, and ears. You can use it in three ways:

- After thumb rolling along for a while, you can stop, maintain pressure on a specific spot, and move the tip of your thumb in very slow circular movements. Move your thumb so it doesn't rub over your skin, but rather moves your skin into and around the underlying tissue.
- When you have been holding a reflex point or area for a time, you can, while maintaining pressure, do the circular movement. Again, don't rub over the skin but slowly move the tissue under the skin around.
- You can go to a reflex point or area and start directly by doing the circular movement. Be sure you're moving the skin and the tissue under the skin, not simply rubbing over it.

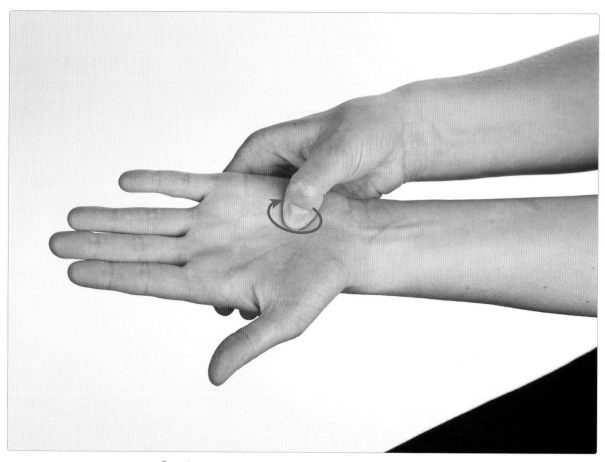

Circular movements one way ...

Remember, go in slow circles. The idea is to break down the underlying chemicals that have accumulated around the nerve endings. Going fast can hurt and can dissipate fewer of the chemicals you want to break down from around the nerve endings.

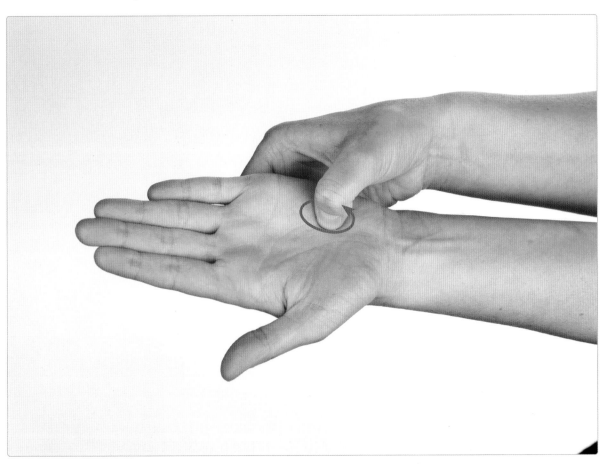

... and circular movements the other way.

Techniques for Ears

When doing reflexology work on your hands and feet, you can only work on one hand or one foot at a time. But with ear reflexology, you can work on both ears at the same time for greater effectiveness and sometimes faster results.

Flowing and holding techniques are the two primary types of reflexing techniques you'll use when working on your ears. When doing an overall session on your ears, start with nurturing flowing techniques and then use holding techniques when you want to reflex for specific issues or certain parts or functions elsewhere in your body.

Flowing techniques help you feel for subtle skin texture differences on and under the skin and in the cartilage of the ear such as bumps, pitted areas, hard or soft tissue or cartilage, and puffiness. Once you become familiar with the different textures and learn what's normal for each part of the ear, you'll be better equipped to notice when you feel unusual textures. For example, if you normally have no unusual neck stress, the neck reflexes in your ear will feel normal. However, if you strain the right half of your neck, you might notice that your ear's neck reflex feels harder than usual and might be slightly tender.

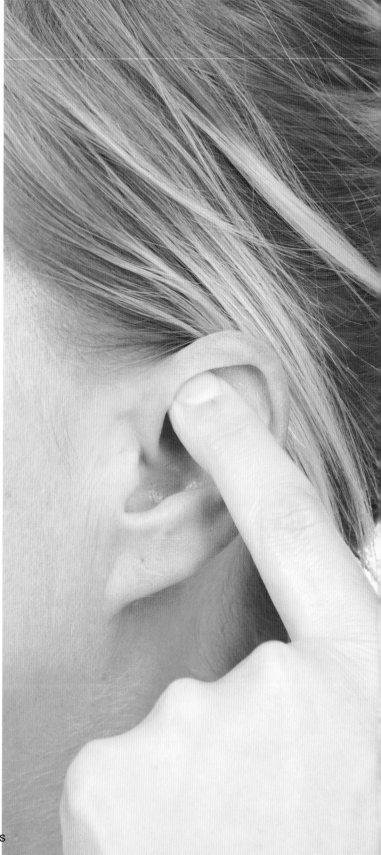

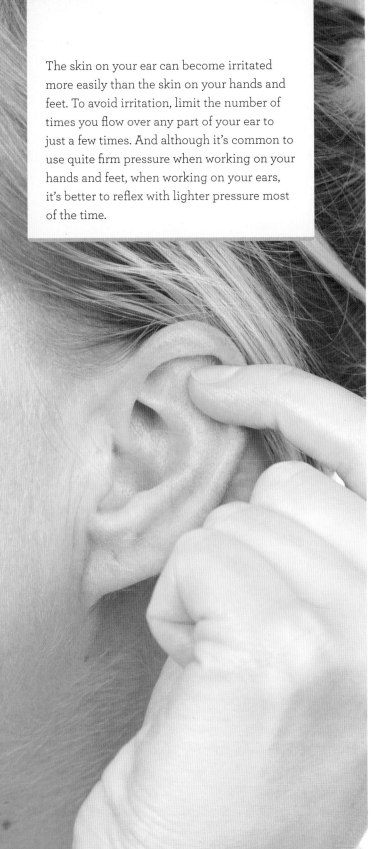

The skin on your ear can become irritated more easily than the skin on your hands and feet. To avoid irritation, limit the number of times you flow over any part of your ear to just a few times. And although it's common to use quite firm pressure when working on your hands and feet, when working on your ears, it's better to reflex with lighter pressure most of the time.

To reflex specific parts of your ears for certain parts or functions of your body, you can use a variety of holding techniques. These techniques enable you to reflex broad areas such as all your neck reflexes or your whole leg reflex. For best results, perform the holding techniques with the softer, fleshier pads of your fingers (usually your index finger) and your thumb. Or you can use your fingertips to target smaller reflexes, such as when you want to focus on only your lower neck reflexes or your knee reflex.

If you've ever had an acupuncture treatment, you might know that acupuncture needles can be left in for anywhere from half an hour to an hour at a time. Although reflexology is quite different from acupuncture, the same principle applies. When working your ears especially, you can hold a reflex for a prolonged period of time, frequently for 5 minutes or more. On some clients with serious health issues, especially pain in other parts of the body, I have held reflexes for as long as 30 minutes or more. You can do the same for yourself. When holding points on your ears, especially for longer spans of time like this, rest your elbows on a table- or desktop to avoid fatiguing your arms and shoulders.

Holding

Holding is an excellent technique to use when reflexing your ears. You can hold in at least six ways: index fingertip, thumb tip, pad to pad, tip to pad, tip to tip, and tip to knuckle. The index and thumb tip holds are best used on parts of the ear you can't get behind, and the others are good for parts you can get behind, such as your earlobe.

When working on your ears, begin with techniques that gently cover broad areas, and then target specific, smaller, reflex areas and points.

How long should you hold? It depends. Sometimes the pain or discomfort goes away in under a minute. At other times, you might have to hold the point longer. See what works best for you in the circumstance.

Index Fingertip Hold

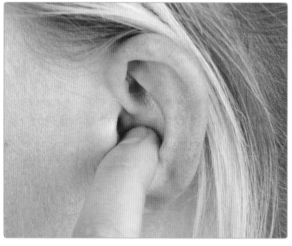

Place tip of your index finger deep into your lower valley, against your head, push against your head, and hold.

Thumb Tip Hold

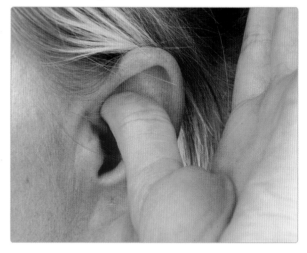

Place the tip of your thumb against your narrow ridge, push against your head, and hold.

Pad-to-Pad Hold

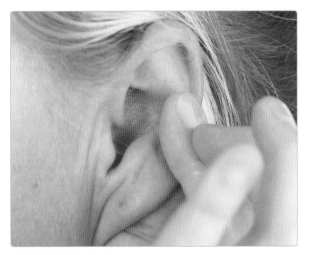

Place the pad of your thumb behind your ear, place the pad of your index finger on the front of the same part of your ear, squeeze, and hold.

Tip-to-Pad Hold

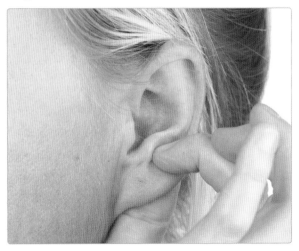

Place the pad of your thumb behind your ear, place the tip of your index finger on the front of the same part of your ear, squeeze, and hold.

Tip-to-Tip Hold

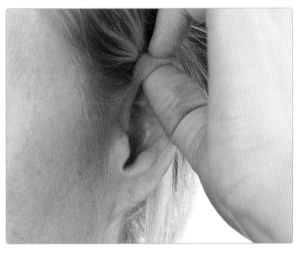

Place the tip of your thumb behind a part of your ear, place the tip of your index finger on the front of the same part of your ear, squeeze (being very attentive to comfort level for your ear), and hold.

Tip-to-Knuckle Hold

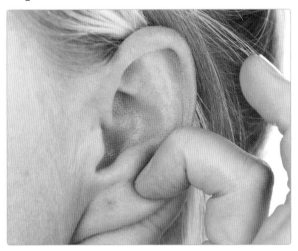

Place the pad of your thumb behind your ear with your thumb's middle knuckle behind the reflex point you want to work. Place the tip of your index finger on the front of the same part of your ear, squeeze carefully, and hold.

Flowing

Flowing movements can feel quite pleasant when you're working on your ears. Flowing, or dragging your fingertip or pad along a reflex area very slowly yet very lightly, lets you feel for slight texture irregularities on and under the skin. Such irregularities can be an indication of possible health issues, current or past, in the related part of the body. Flowing very slowly but firmly can help you break down chemicals around the nerve endings in the reflexes you're flowing over.

Only flow in one direction. Because it can feel irritating, don't flow back and forth.

Flowing with Your Fingertip Against Your Ear

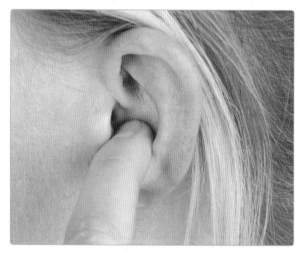

Place the tip of your index finger deep into your lower valley, near your ear canal, and push against your head. Bring your finger straight back for a few centimeters. Lift your fingertip, return to the starting place, and repeat.

Flowing with the Tip of Your Thumb Against Your Ear's Outer Ridge

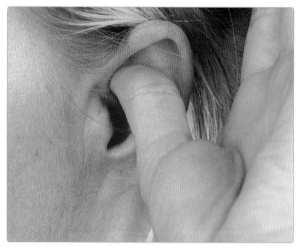

Place the tip of your thumb against the root of your outer ridge, push against your head, and flow in one direction. Repeat.

Flowing with the Tip of Your Finger

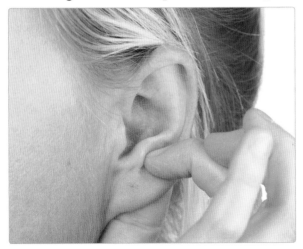

Place the pad of your thumb behind your ear, and place the tip of your index finger on the front of the same part of your ear. Squeeze and flow with your index finger, maintaining gentle pressure. Repeat flowing in the same direction.

Flowing with the Pad of Your Finger

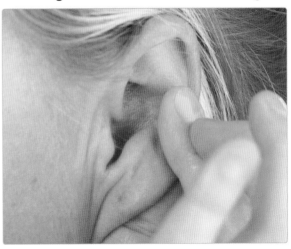

Place the pad of your thumb behind your ear, and place the pad of your index finger on the front of the same part of your ear. Squeeze and flow with your index finger, maintaining gentle pressure. Repeat flowing in the same direction.

Flowing with the Tip of Your Thumb

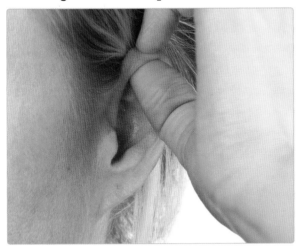

Place the pad of your index finger behind your ear, and place the tip of your thumb on the front of the same part of your ear. Squeeze and flow with your thumb, maintaining gentle pressure. Repeat flowing in the same direction.

Flowing with the Pad of Your Thumb

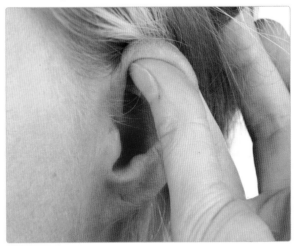

Place the pad of your index finger behind your ear, and place the pad of your thumb on the front of the same part of your ear. Squeeze and flow with your thumb, maintaining gentle pressure. Repeat flowing in the same direction.

Applying Pressure

One of the most common questions people have when they begin reflexology, on themselves or on a loved one, is how much pressure to apply while they're working. The answer is, it depends.

Every person is different, and what one person feels is pleasant pressure versus unpleasant differs as well. What's more, the levels of pressure that might feel good or uncomfortable on your foot might not be the same as on your hand, which might not be the same as on your ear.

Tenderness and Sensitivity

As you do reflexology for a while, you'll discover that the degree of tenderness or sensitivity for each part of the foot, hand, or ear varies from day to day and week to week, depending on a wide range of factors, such as your diet, exercise level—even the weather! Generally speaking, depending on the techniques you use, your feet tend to be a bit more sensitive, your hands are a little less sensitive, and your ears are even less sensitive.

When working on yourself, you have the advantage of feeling what amount of pressure is pleasant versus unpleasant on each part, and you can regulate the amount of pressure you apply. If you like deeper pressure, you you can work at that level. If you prefer lighter pressure, you can make that accommodation.

Think about the last time somebody massaged your shoulders. At some point, you might have said "Ouch," but quickly followed that with "Please don't stop," especially if the masseuse pulled away his or her hands. There can be a pleasant level of tenderness that's quite acceptable, and you're likely to experience this as you practice reflexology. Most of the time, reflexology should feel pleasant, so use the amount of pressure that either causes no tenderness or is on the pleasant side of tenderness.

Do not work at a level of pressure that causes pain or discomfort. You don't want to cause yourself or anyone else pain, and excessive tenderness can be counterproductive to your body's healing process.

If you're new to reflexology, the first few times you work on your feet, hands, and ears, do so on the lighter side of tenderness. This way, you won't strain your hands and thumbs and you'll detox slowly, breaking down the irritating chemicals around the nerve endings gradually. Use lighter pressure at first, working between the soft surface tissue and firmer deeper tissue, and the deeper tissue will start to soften. Soon you'll be able to go deeper without using more pressure with your thumbs and hands, which will keep you from straining your hands and thumbs.

Working on Someone Else

When you reflex someone else, all the same principles apply. The main difference is that you need to communicate with the recipient and ask for their feedback so you can learn what level of pressure is pleasant or unpleasant for them.

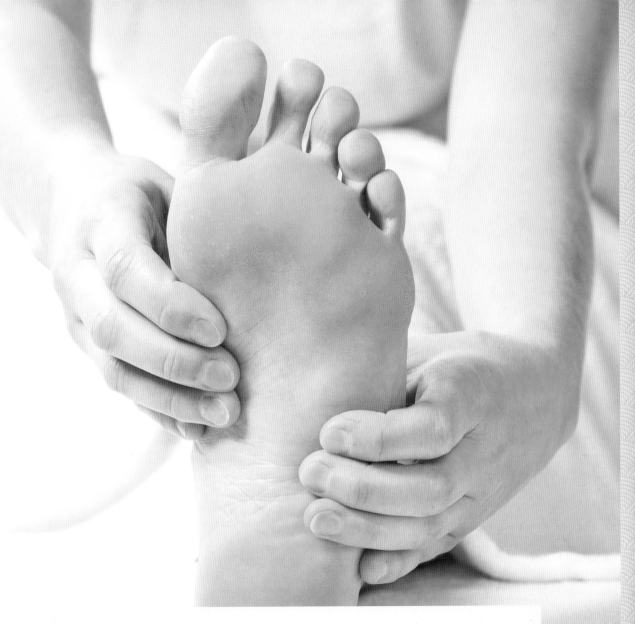

When you find tenderness in your feet, hands, or ears, think of it as a gift—as your body's way of asking you to pay attention to something. Although the tenderness might be because of a current or past aliment or issue in the related part of your body, it could also be because of a current or past strain, stress, or trauma in your feet, hands, or ears. For example, you might have twisted your ankle sometime in the past, strained your hand opening a jar, or slept with your ear folded under. So when you apply pressure and find tenderness in your feet, hands, or ears, consider it an opportunity to use reflexology to help your body heal the issues in the related part or right where you're touching.

Helpful Reflexology Tools

As you've learned, you don't really need any tools or equipment to perform reflexology, but some tools might come in handy from time to time as you reflex your own feet and hands.

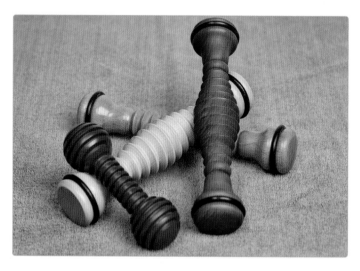

The Roller

One of the most common reflexology tools is the *foot roller* or *reflexology roller*. Rollers are most often made of wood or plastic; can range in size from 6 to 12 inches (15 to 30cm) wide; and contain a variety of types of ridges, grooves, bumps, and protrusions.

If you're new to using rollers, you might want to start by wearing a thick sock for more padding and using the foot roller while you're sitting down so you exert less pressure on it.

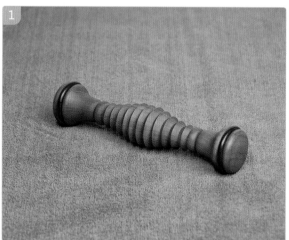

Place the roller on the floor in front of you, preferably on a carpeted floor.

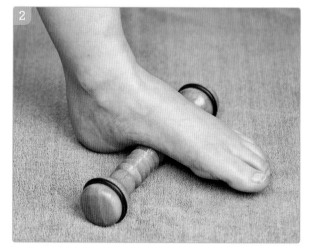

Set your foot on top of the roller, apply gentle pressure, and slowly roll your foot back and forth so you provide enough time to break down the irritating chemicals around nerve endings in the reflex areas on your feet.

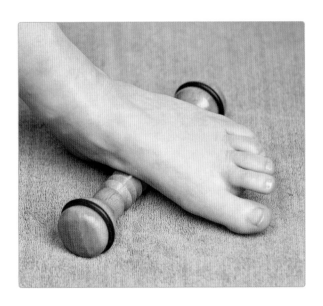

You might find some of the tools discussed in this section beneficial when you're reflexing your own feet and hands, but they're not recommended for use when you're giving someone else reflexology. The tools don't give you the same sense of touch, of feeling, as your fingers. You won't be as able to tell, for example, when you've used too much pressure or hit a sensitive spot. It's best, therefore, to use these tools only when doing reflexology work on yourself and not on others.

Instead of rolling, you also can apply direct pressure to one specific spot you want to target, such as the arch of your foot.

The same roller also is very versatile for reflexing your hands. There are two main ways to use rollers for your hands:

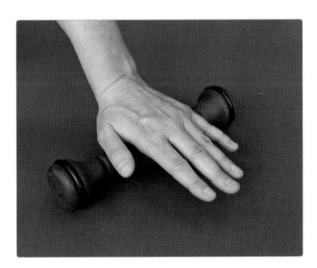

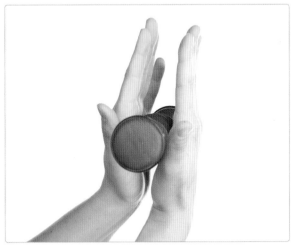

Place the roller on a desk- or tabletop; set your hand on top of the roller; and apply gentle pressure with your palm, the inner edge of your hand, or the outer edge of your hand. Either keep your hand on the roller on one specific spot you want to target, or roll your hand back and forth very slowly.

You also could clasp the roller between the palms of your hands, squeeze, and roll slowly back and forth. Intertwining your fingers can help you get a firmer squeeze.

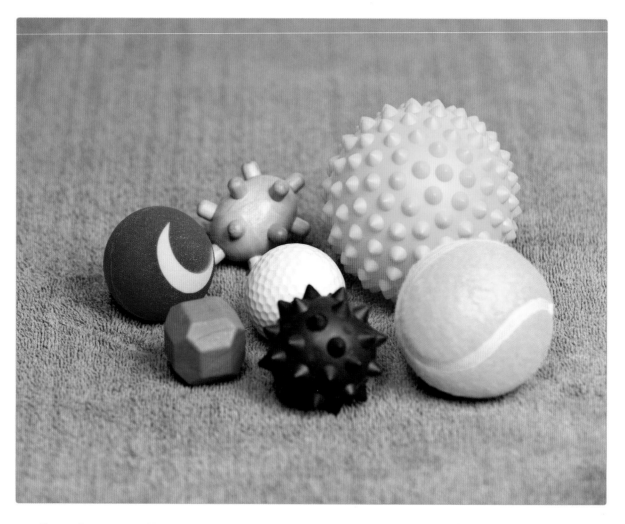

Reflexology Balls

Many variations of *reflexology balls* are available to use when you're treating yourself to reflexology. They can be made of wood, plastic, stone, metal, buffalo horns, and other materials. They can vary in size and texture, too. Some have ridges, grooves, bumps, circular indentations, and slight to extreme protrusions.

But with all the fancier reflexology balls available, the most commonly used ball during reflexology sessions is a golf ball. You can use a golf ball on your feet as well as your hands.

One year when I was flying around the world on a reflexology teaching tour (I was in 65 airplanes that year!), I would, upon arriving in a new city, walk around town until I found a round stone to roll my feet with each morning and evening.

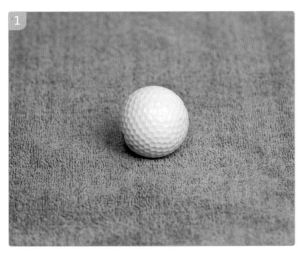

Place the golf ball on the floor, preferably on a carpet so it doesn't slide around.

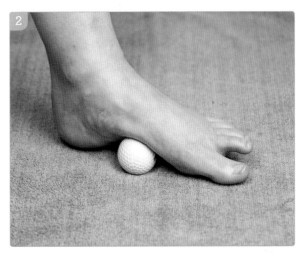

Set your foot on top of the ball, apply gentle pressure, and slowly roll your foot in various directions so you allow enough time to break down the irritating chemicals around nerve endings in the reflex areas on your feet.

Here are two ways to use a golf ball during a hand reflexology routine:

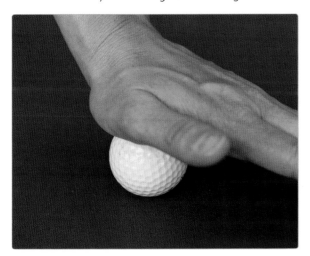

Place the golf ball on a desk- or tabletop, set your hand on top of the ball, and apply gentle pressure with your palm. Either keep your hand on the ball on one specific spot, or roll your hand very slowly.

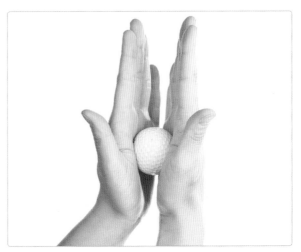

Or clasp the golf ball between your palms, squeeze, and roll slowly in circular movements. Intertwine your fingers for a firmer squeeze.

A Few More Pointers

Now that you've learned the specific techniques you'll use when reflexing your own feet, hands, and ears, you still might have some questions. Let's go over a few more points of interest before we end this part of the book.

How Long Should I Work?

When you're doing full foot, hand, or ear reflexology routines on yourself, keep the session to between 30 and 45 minutes.

When you're working on specific reflexes for specific parts of your body, how long you work on that reflex point or area depends on a number of factors. For example, when you're working to relieve a long-term issue, such as chronic shoulder joint pain, consider working on your shoulder joint reflexes on your feet for 10 to 15 minutes. Then move to your hands and work for 10 to 15 more minutes. Finish by working on your ears for a final 10 to 15 minutes.

If you're in severe pain, such as when you have a migraine or horrible headache, you can work on the brain reflexes on your feet, hands, and ears as well as the big web of your hand, between your thumb and the rest of your hand, for 30 minutes, 60 minutes, or more.

If you do work for long periods of time on one reflex point or area, start by using lighter pressure and gradually increasing how hard you push and how deep you go into the tissue.

In any one situation, you might have 5 or 10 minutes to work on your feet, hands, and ears. Other times, you might have an hour. Use whatever time you have available to make the most of your reflexology work to achieve the most benefits.

Which Area Should I Work?

If you're wondering which area you should work for maximum benefit, I'll let you in on a little secret: work all three—your feet, hands, and ears—for the best results.

Each area has unique advantages, and each has specific conditions or issues for which it's most effective. Working on all three areas during the same session yields better results than if you only working on one or two areas.

Throughout the book, and especially with the ailments, I've often suggested where to work first and how to progress from there. Sometimes I specifically call out two of the three, but that doesn't mean you work those two areas and then omit the third. For best results, go ahead and do the third as well.

Remember the importance of drinking extra water to help flush out toxins that are likely to be released during a longer reflexology session.

Which Side Do I Reflex?

The text and photo instructions throughout the book focus on the left foot, the left hand, and the left ear unless otherwise indicated. These instructions are the same for the right foot, hand, and ear, so just switch sides when you're done with your left side. Note, however, that some reflex areas are only on the left side or only on the right side; I point out those areas in the text.

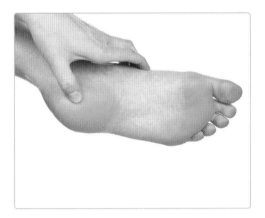

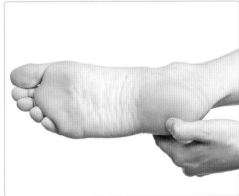

Pay attention to the text and watch the photos to see which side of your body should be reflexing.

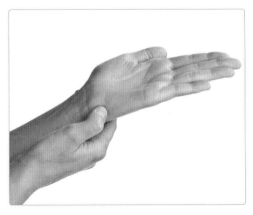

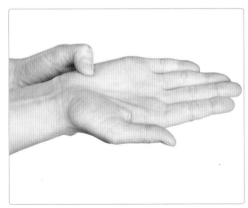

Is There Any Difference When Working on Someone Else?

Throughout the book, the directions are written and the photos show each technique from your viewpoint so you can learn how to reflex your own feet, hands, and ears. If you're performing reflexology on someone else, simply adapt the directions as necessary.

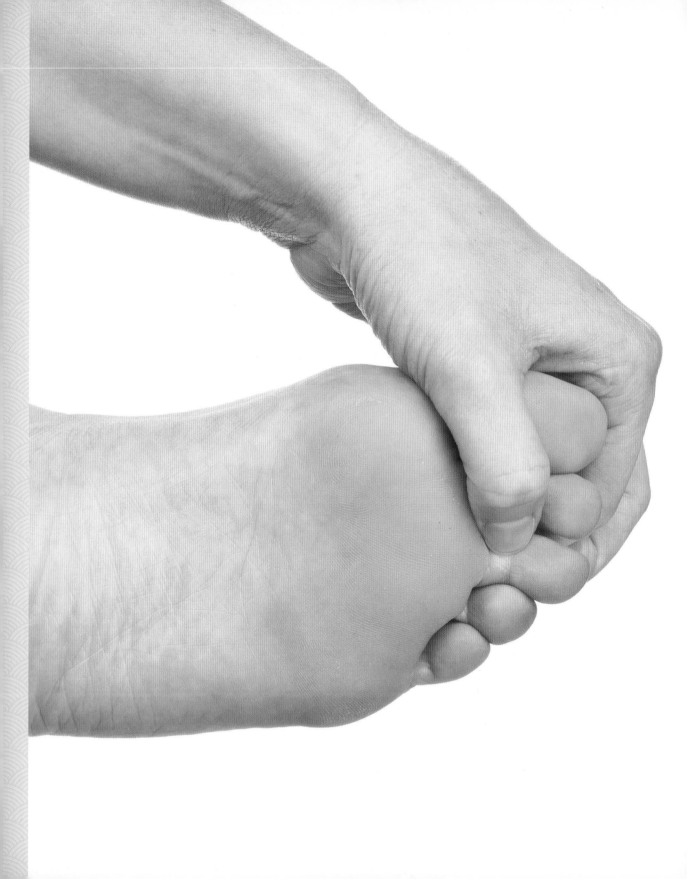

Part 4

Reflexology for the Feet

Many people find a foot rub relaxing. However, as you learn throughout this book, reflexology is very different from a simple foot rub and not only can be relaxing, but can also help your body heal itself. To perform reflexology well, you need to know the geography of the reflex points and areas on the feet as well as how to best touch those spots for the most healing benefits throughout your body. In this part, you learn the topography of the foot's reflex areas and how to combine them into a 1-hour foot reflexology routine. By reflexing your feet completely, you not only help the place where you feel the pain or discomfort, but you also make better the source of your pain elsewhere in your body.

The Bottoms of the Toes

Your brain affects the health of your entire body. Your pituitary gland, nestled in the middle of your brain, releases chemicals that affect glands in other parts of your body. Those glands, in turn, impact your overall health and well-being.

The muscles at the top of your neck connect into your head, and at the bottom of your neck, they connect to your upper back, your shoulders, and your chest. As your neck relaxes, it not only helps ease pain and discomforts in your neck but also helps relax most of your head, chest, and shoulders.

Your big toe is home to the reflex points for your head and neck. The longer you work on your big toes, the more benefits you reap in this area that all too easily holds onto stress and other issues.

Your left big toe is home to reflexes for everything in the left half of your head and neck, and your right toe holds reflexes for the right half of your head and neck. By working on both big toes completely, you reflex for everything in this area.

The tip of your big toe equates to the top of your head. The middle joint of your big toe is more for the bottom of your head or top of your neck. The bottom of your big toe is for the bottom of your neck.

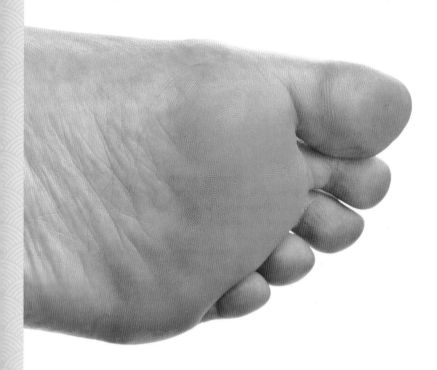

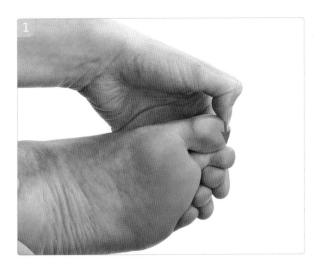

Place your thumb on the outside edge of the bottom side surface of your big toe, near the tip, and reflex across your toe.

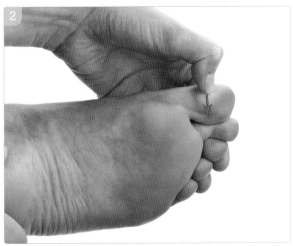

Thumb roll across your toe, including the middle knuckle. Overlap as you work across, moving a little lower on your toe each time.

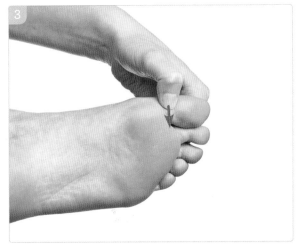

Continue thumb rolling across your big toe's bottom side surface until you reach the base where your toe joins your foot.

The Bottoms of the Toes *(continued)*

In addition to working the bottom side of your big toes, you can reflex the bottom of your other toes as well. Your four smaller toes are also linked to your head and neck, making them ideal for reflexing for head and neck issues.

Closer to the tip of your toes is for your upper head and brain. The middle part of your toes is more for your lower head and upper neck. Close to the bottom of your toes corresponds to your middle and lower neck.

Usually, it feels quite nice to reflex your own toes or have someone reflex them for you. However, you can experience some discomfort or even pain when you begin to work on your four smaller toes.

Start reflexing the bottoms of your toes with light pressure, using the pad of your thumb. If you don't experience any discomfort, and if you'd like to work more deeply, you can gradually apply more pressure with the pad of your thumb. Or if you'd like to do more detailed reflexing, getting into smaller, more targeted spots, you can use more of the tip of your thumb.

For some people, the bottom surface of the big toe can be quite soft. If yours is, apply lighter pressure at first as you reflex. If that pressure is still too much or causes you any pain, work even lighter.

On the other hand, some people have very hard or callused tissue on the bottom side surface of their big toes. If yours is hard, apply pressure that's pleasantly firm yet not firm enough to cause discomfort to either your toe or your reflexing hand or thumb.

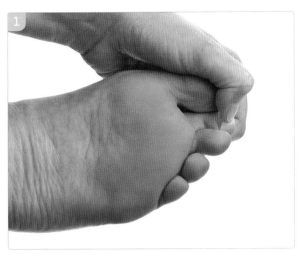

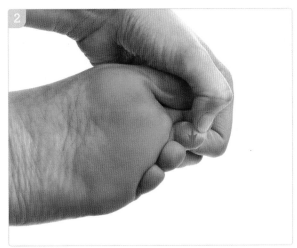

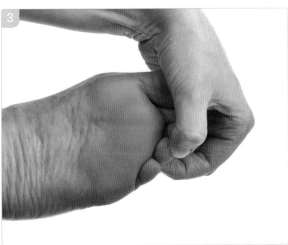

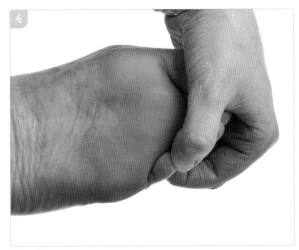

When reflexing your smaller toes, place the pad of your thumb on the bottom side of your toe, near the tip, and thumb roll across your toes, overlapping as you work across, moving a little lower on your toe each time.

The Tops of the Toes

Reflexing the tops of your toes can be helpful for easing discomforts in your head and neck, similar to working the bottoms of your toes. Reflexing on top of your big toe, for example, near the nail can be especially helpful for easing dental pain and sore gums. Reflex closer to the tips of your toes for issues with your upper head and brain. The middle part of your toes corresponds more to your lower head and upper neck. Closer toward the base of your toes aligns with your middle and lower neck.

When working on your big toe, place the pad of your index finger on top of your toe, just below your toenail, and do an index finger roll to the base of your toe where it joins your foot.

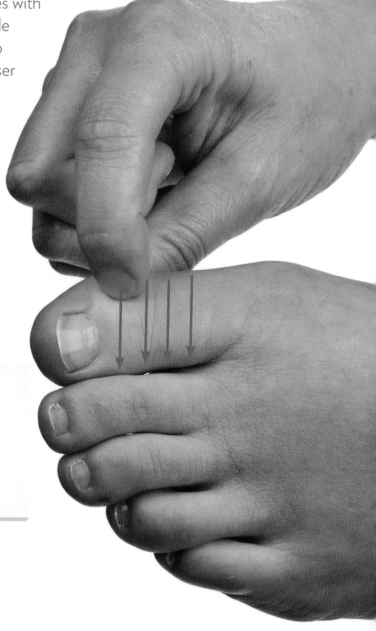

Working on the tops of your own toes can be awkward for some people. It helps if you sit with your working leg bent and resting on your other knee. The closer your foot is to your knee, the easier it should be to reach your foot for reflexology work.

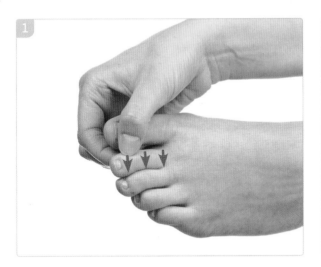

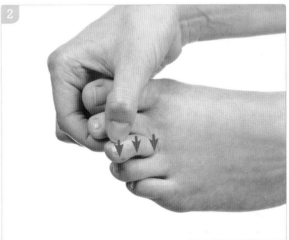

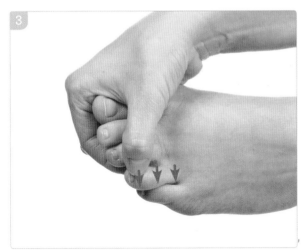

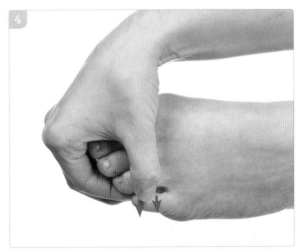

When reflexing your smaller toes, place the tip of your index finger on top of your toe, just below your nail, and do an index finger roll to the base of your toe where it joins your foot. You also could use your thumb.

The Outer Sides of the Toes

Working on the outer sides on your own toes can be a little awkward for some people, but reflexing this area is so valuable, especially if you have head, neck, or sinus issues.

Reflexing the outer sides of your toes can be helpful for easing discomforts in your head and neck, especially sinus issues. The area closer to the tips of your toes corresponds to your upper head and brain. The middle parts of your toes are more for your lower head and upper neck. The base of your toes, where they join your foot, aligns with your middle and lower neck.

When working on your big toe, place the pad of your index finger between your big toe and your second toe so you're touching the side of your big toe. Starting near the tip of your big toe, do an index finger roll from near the tip all the way down to the base of your toe where it joins your foot. Repeat several times to get all parts of that outer side of your big toe.

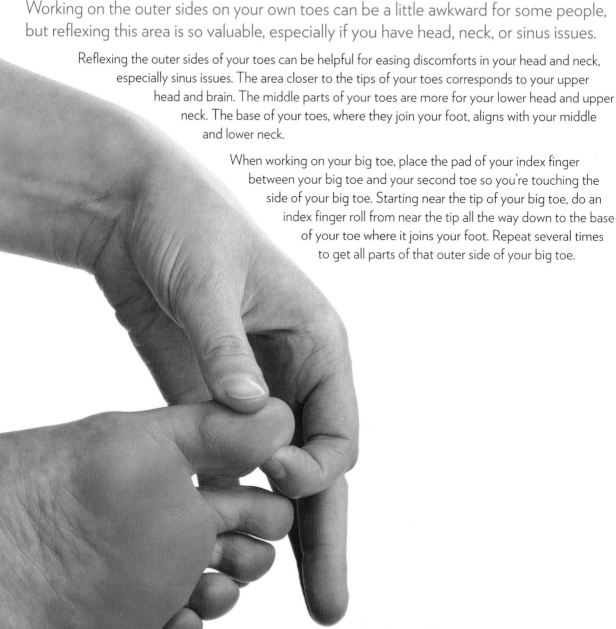

Reflex closer to the tips of your toes for relief of upper sinus issues, work midway down your toe for middle- and lower-sinus issues, and concentrate on the lower part of your toes to relax your neck, which also helps relax your sinuses.

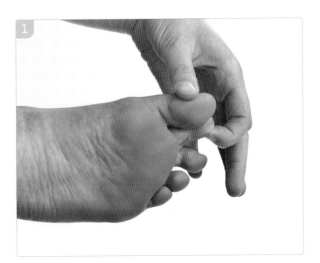

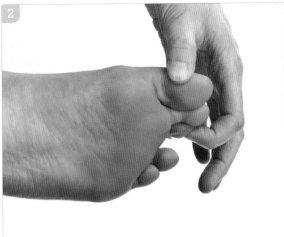

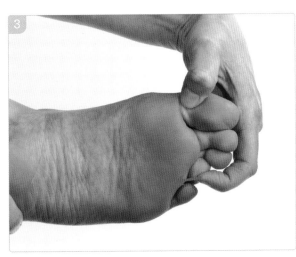

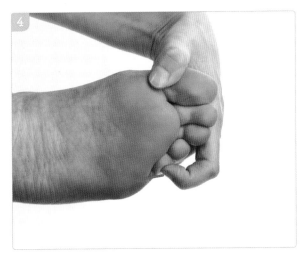

When reflexing your smaller toes, place the pad of your index finger on the outer side of your toe, near the tip. Do an index finger roll from near the tip to the base of your toe, where it joins your foot.

The Inner Sides of the Toes

Fortunately, working on the inner sides on your toes can be a lot easier than working on the outer sides.

Reflexing the inner sides of your toes can be helpful for easing discomforts in your head and neck, especially sinus issues. Working closer to the tip of your toes helps your upper head and brain. Reflexing the middle part of your toes benefits your lower head and upper neck. Working close toward the bottom of your toes aligns with your middle and lower neck.

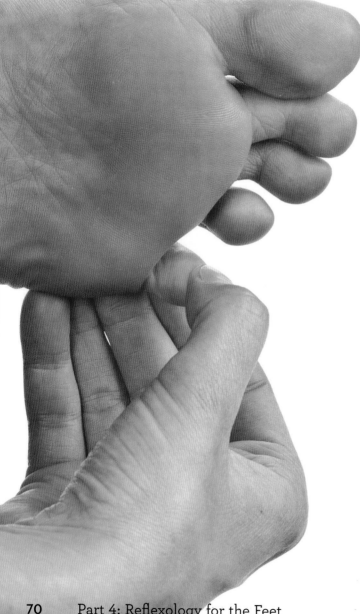

Reflex closer to the tip of the inner sides of your toes for upper sinus relief, work midway down your toes for middle and lower sinus issues, and focus on the lower part of your toes to relax your neck, which also helps relax your sinuses.

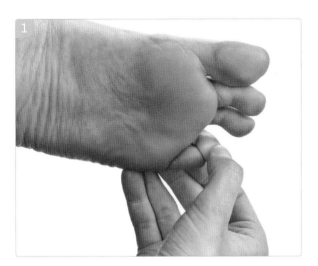

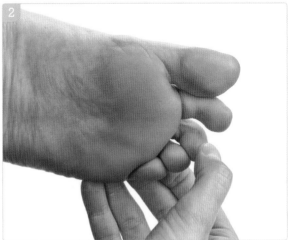

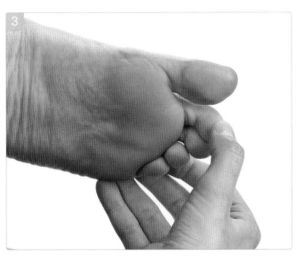

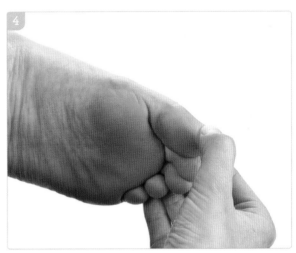

When reflexing your toes, place the pad of your thumb on the inner side of your toe, near the tip. Do a thumb roll from near the tip to the base of your toe where it joins your foot.

The Ball and Pad of the Foot

The ball and pad of your foot is the area located between the base of your toes and your arch—it's where your toes connect with your foot. People who frequently wear higher-heeled shoes or sharp, pointed shoes can experience foot discomfort and pain in this area.

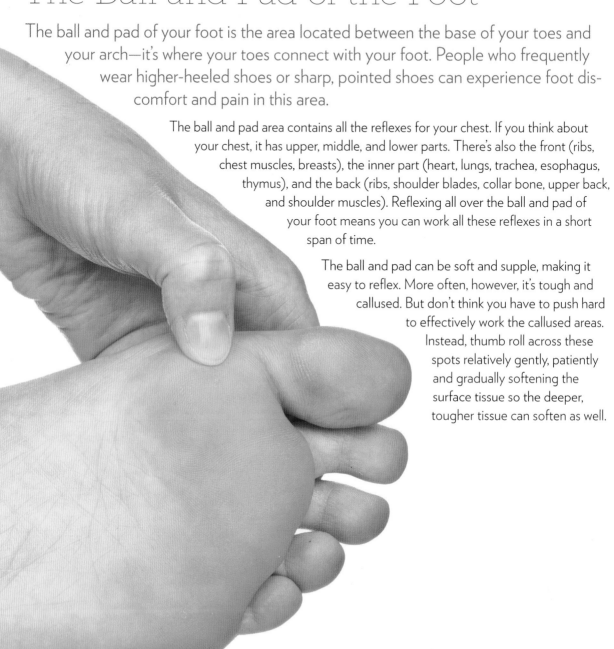

The ball and pad area contains all the reflexes for your chest. If you think about your chest, it has upper, middle, and lower parts. There's also the front (ribs, chest muscles, breasts), the inner part (heart, lungs, trachea, esophagus, thymus), and the back (ribs, shoulder blades, collar bone, upper back, and shoulder muscles). Reflexing all over the ball and pad of your foot means you can work all these reflexes in a short span of time.

The ball and pad can be soft and supple, making it easy to reflex. More often, however, it's tough and callused. But don't think you have to push hard to effectively work the callused areas. Instead, thumb roll across these spots relatively gently, patiently and gradually softening the surface tissue so the deeper, tougher tissue can soften as well.

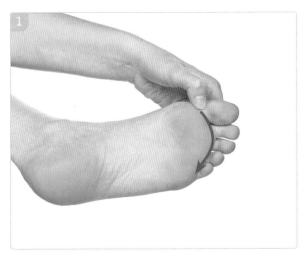

On the ball of your foot, just below the base of your big toe, thumb roll across the pad of your foot to just below your small toe.

At some point in your life, you might have twisted your ankle. Sometimes a severe twist can force some of the ankle bones out of alignment, which can force the long bones of your foot out of alignment, too. The effect can be seen on the pad, where a callous under the head of the second, third, or fourth long bone develops. Reflexology can minimize and sometimes eliminate pain and discomfort related to this issue, but prevention by wearing smarter shoes or correction by a podiatrist is probably best.

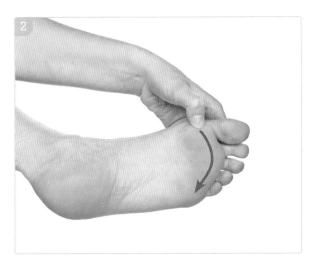

Repeat thumb rolling across the ball and pad of your foot, each time going across a little more toward the heel, overlapping a little each time you go across.

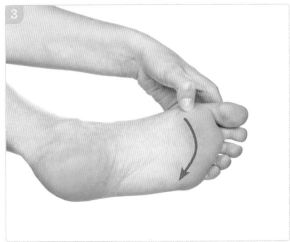

Continue overlapping, as you thumb roll across your foot, row by row.

Spend extra time going across the bottom of your ball and pad, the part close to your arch.

The Arch

Your arch makes up a relatively large part of the bottom of your foot, and much of it is rather soft, especially the surface tissue.

The arch of your foot is home to reflexes for your upper abdomen. On the left side are reflexes for your stomach, a lobe of your liver, your spleen, the body and tail of your pancreas, your left kidney and adrenal gland, and part of your colon. On the right are reflexes for your liver, gallbladder, common bile duct, the head of your pancreas, your right kidney and adrenal gland, and another part of your colon. The inner edge holds reflexes for your middle and lower spinal column and spinal cord.

Reflexing across the upper part of your arch near your ball and pad for several minutes a day can gradually soften the deeper muscles in your arch and dramatically reduce upper-abdominal discomforts such as upset stomach, stomach cramps, nausea, and gallstone pain. Reflexing across the rest of your arch can help with colon issues such as constipation, diarrhea, gas pains, and more.

In contrast to how tough the ball and pad and heel of your foot can be, your arch's surface layer of tissue can be quite soft. The deeper layers, closer to the bones, are usually much tighter. As you work, use your nonreflexing hand to gently bend your toes toward your heel. This softens the deeper, tighter muscles in the area, enabling you to better reflex your arch without having to push harder to get into the deeper tissue.

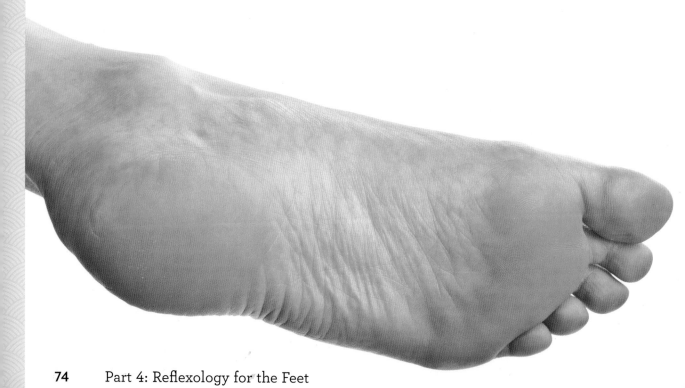

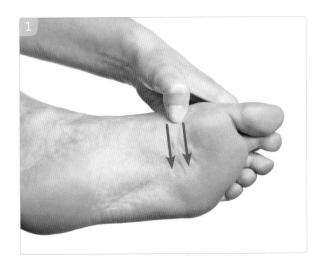

If you have pain in your abdominal muscles from activities such as coughing too much or doing abdominal crunches, you can find some relief by reflexing your arch.

Place your thumb on the inner edge of your arch, near your ball and pad. Thumb roll across your arch, from the inner edge to the outer edge.

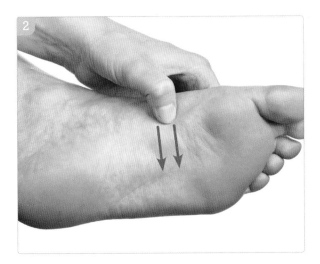

Move your starting point a little closer to your heel, and thumb roll across your arch again, overlapping a little each time you go across.

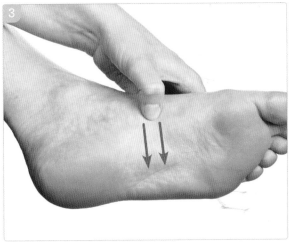

Continue overlapping as you go across, row by row, thumb rolling across your arch until you're near your heel.

The Heel

Your heel is the first part of your foot to touch the ground when you walk. Because of this important role, the skin on your heel can be quite tough and even callused, making it difficult to reflex.

Your heel holds reflexes for your lower abdominal area and pelvis, both internally (your lower small intestines, ileocecal valve, appendix, lower colon, reproductive system, urinary bladder, and more) and external (your pelvic muscles, pelvic girdle muscles, and buttock muscles), as well as your pelvic bones..

You might be tempted to skip reflexing your heel if you have especially tough skin there. I encourage you to work on your heel anyway because it's an important area for relaxation and increased circulation for your lower abdomen and entire pelvic musculature. Don't push hard as you reflex. Instead, thumb roll across your heel relatively gently, slowly softening the surface tissue so the deeper tissue below also can soften.

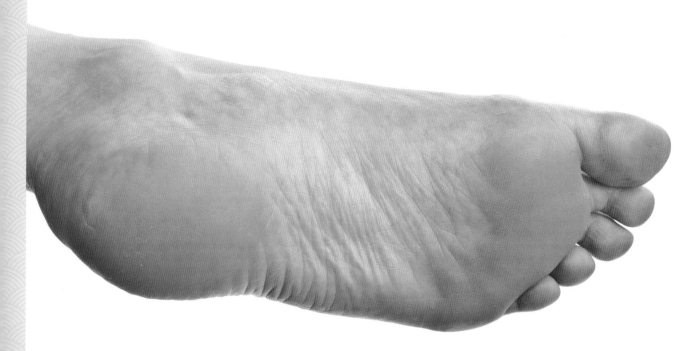

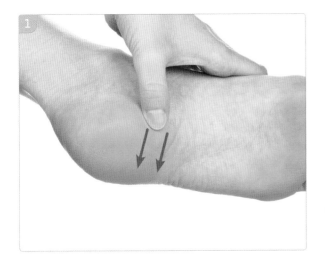

A fair number of people have heel spurs or plantar fasciitis. If you do, use light pressure when reflexing, use the pad of your thumb, and work for short periods of time—say, 5 to 10 minutes if possible every other day or so.

Place your thumb at the inner edge of your heel, near your arch. Thumb roll across from the outer edge of your heel to the inner edge, near your arch.

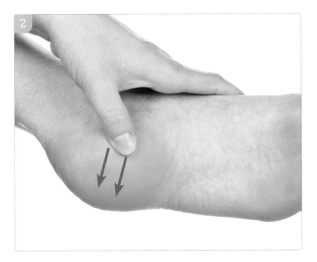

Move your starting point a little closer to the back of your foot, and thumb roll across your heel again, overlapping a little each time you go across.

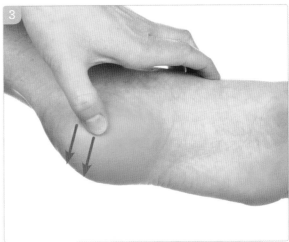

Continue overlapping as you go across your heel, row by row, thumb rolling across until you've covered your whole heel.

The Outer Edge of the Foot and the Back of the Heel

The outer edge of the foot is often overlooked when it comes to at-home reflexology sessions. And that's a shame! This area is home to reflex areas for everything from your upper arms to your fingertips, and from your hips to the tips of your toes. By reflexing this area, you reflex for the entire side of your torso and, when you work down near your heel, for your reproductive health, too.

The outer edge of your foot, from the bottom of your little toe almost to your heel, contains reflexes for your entire upper arm, elbow, forearm, wrist, hands, and fingers. The area from the soft triangle below and in front of your ankle bone, to your heel, and to the base of your Achilles tendon is home to reflexes for your hip, upper leg, knee, lower leg, ankle, foot, and toes.

The area behind the heel bone has been helpful for easing hemorrhoid discomforts. Reflexing the back of your heel a couple times a day can be helpful for preventing, or at least minimizing, such discomforts.

Most of the blood in your body is produced in the long and flat bones in your body. The outer edge of your foot contains reflexes for most of your long bones and some of your flat bones.

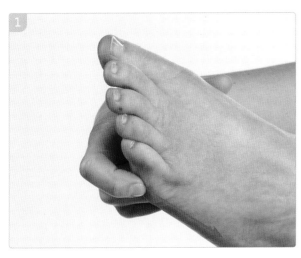

Place the tip of your index finger on the outer edge of your foot, below your little toe, and do an index finger roll.

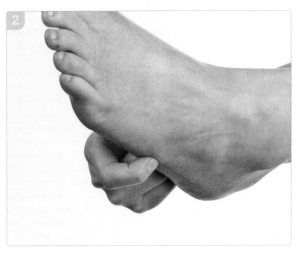

Continue using an index finger roll with the tip of your finger, down the outer edge of your foot, all the way to your heel.

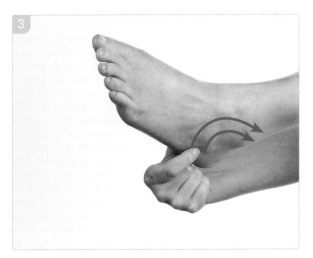

Reflex the entire area below your outer ankle bone, all the way back to your heel, and to the base of your Achilles tendon.

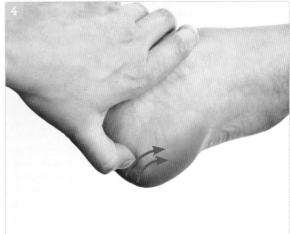

Finally, thumb roll all over the back of your heel bone.

The Outer Edge of the Foot and the Back of the Heel 　79

The Inner Edge of the Foot

The inner edge of your foot is a valuable area to reflex for the health of your spinal column—really, the health of your entire body. From each set of bones in your spinal column, peripheral nerves radiate out to organs, glands, and structures throughout your body. By reflexing the inner edge of your foot and, therefore, your spinal column, you provide benefits for so much more.

The inner edge of the foot contains a variety of reflexes. Starting near your inner ankle, you have the uterus and prostate reflexes; your heel near the bottom of your foot has your tailbone and sacrum reflexes; the inner edge of your arch near your heel has your lumbar and sciatic nerve reflexes; and along the inner edge of the long bone below your big toes are your thoracic to mid spinal cord and spinal column reflexes.

When you have tension in your spinal muscles—and many people do have tightness in those muscles—the bioelectric flow is reduced between your spinal cord and the related parts of your body. The longer this flow is reduced, the greater the chance organs, glands, and structures throughout your body will start to falter and eventually even malfunction.

Even if you don't feel any spinal pain or discomfort, it's wise to frequently reflex the inner edge of your feet to help reduce long-term tension and permit more optimal bioelectric flow throughout your body.

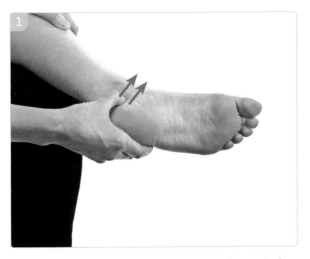

Grasp the outer side of your heel, place the pad of your thumb on the inner side of your heel, and reflex your entire inner ankle with a thumb roll.

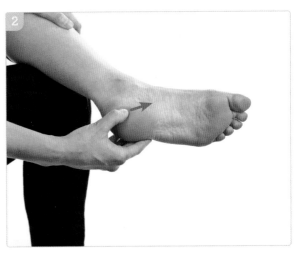

Focus your thumb roll on the inner edge of your heel, closest to the sole of your foot.

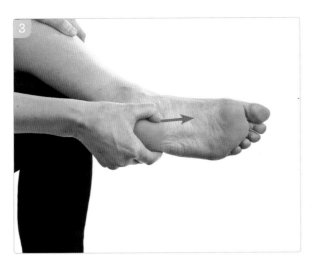

Thumb roll on the inner edge of your foot, closest to your arch, right near your heel.

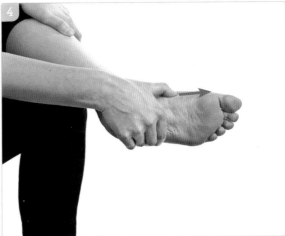

Thumb roll against the inner edge of your long bone, move to the groove slightly on the arch side of that bone, and then work on the inner edge of the muscle on the bottom of your foot.

Avoid working your inner ankle if you're in your first trimester of pregnancy.

The Top of the Foot

The top of your foot is a wonderful area to reflex if you have issues in your chest, such as respiratory problems, or shoulder-related pain.

The top of the foot is home to a multitude of reflexes: those for the front of your chest, including your chest muscles, breasts, and ribs; your inner chest—your heart, lungs, trachea, esophagus, and thymus; and the area behind your chest—your ribs, upper back muscles, collarbone, shoulder blade, the muscles between your shoulder blades, and your shoulder joint.

The chest is an area where many people hold tension, which can contribute to tightening muscles. Tight chest muscles lead to shallow breathing, with less oxygen taken into the lungs, absorbed into the blood, taken to the body, and distributed to all your body's cells. Reflexing the grooves on the top of your foot on a regular basis (perhaps once or twice each day) can help those muscles relax, providing more oxygen to your cells, helping every cell work better, and boosting your overall health, well-being, and vitality.

If you have tight shoulders, shoulder discomfort, or pain in your shoulder joint, reflexing the grooves on top of your feet once or twice a day can provide some relief for these issues as well.

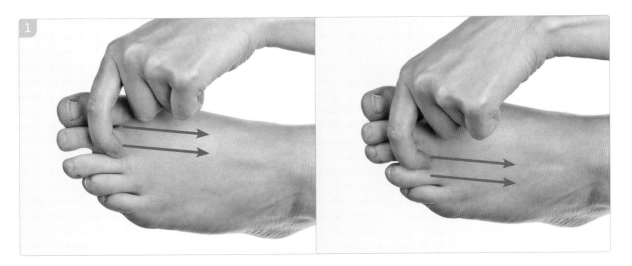

Grasp your arch with your thumb, place the tip of your index finger in the web between your big toe and your second toe, and do a sideways index finger roll in the web and between the joints. Repeat for the webs between your remaining toes.

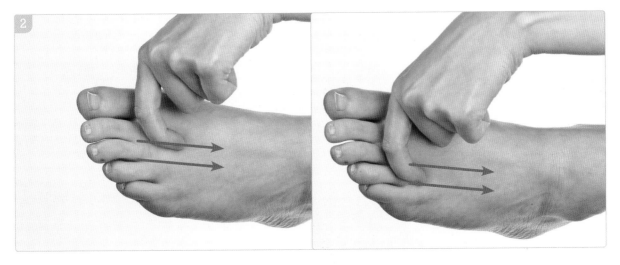

Grasp your arch with your thumb, place the tip of your index finger in the first groove on top of your foot, and do a sideways index finger roll. Repeat in the second, third, and fourth groove.

The Ankle

Look at the lower part of your leg, where it connects with the top of your foot. As you flex your foot up, notice the crease that forms there, between your lower leg and your foot. That's your ankle groove. When your foot is relaxed, you can reflex into that ankle groove.

This area contains the reflexes for the female fallopian tubes (oviducts), the male vas deferens (sperm ducts), as well as the muscles and lymph nodes for the groin.

Reflexing the ankle helps increase circulation in these areas and can help lessen the pain caused by sports injuries, sprains, and strains in the groin. In addition, it has been known to improve circulation and reduce and eliminate inflammation and pain in the groin lymph nodes.

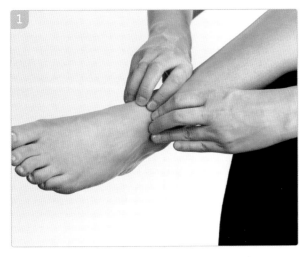

Remember, you'll be able to get into your ankle groove better when your foot is relaxed. If your foot is pointed downward, the groove becomes too tight to reflex. If your foot is flexed toward your leg, the groove becomes too narrow to be able to get into very deeply. The more relaxed you ankle is, the better.

Place the tips of the index, middle, and ring fingers of both hands firmly in your ankle groove. Hold for 5 second and then release. Repeat several times.

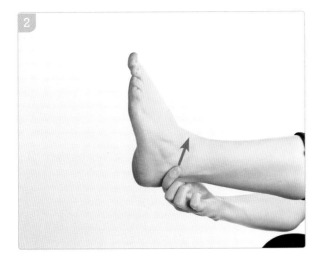

Index finger roll between the center of your ankle groove and your outer ankle bone.

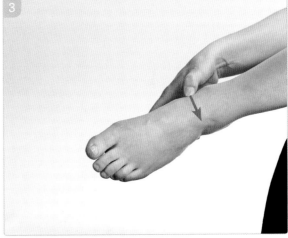

Thumb roll between your inner ankle bone and the center of your ankle groove.

Relaxation Techniques for the Feet

Reflexology in general is relaxing, but sometimes you need a bit more pampering for your feet, especially after a reflexology session or other foot-tiring event. These relaxation techniques are designed to help improve mobility and circulation in different parts of your feet—and feel good while doing so!

For each of these relaxation techniques, we've shown the left foot being worked. Be sure to switch to your right foot for equal relaxation time!

The Foot Flip

The foot flip can help relax the muscles, ligaments, and tendons in your ankles, as well as improve circulation throughout most of your foot. This helps increase your range of motion in your feet.

The first few times you try this relaxation technique, you might find letting your ankle and foot relax a bit challenging. But stick with it—it's worth it!

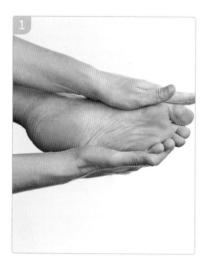 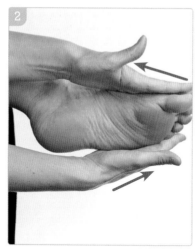 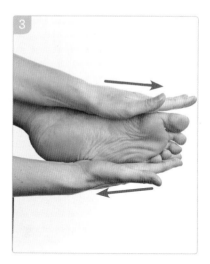

Place the palm of your right hand against the outer edge of your foot and the palm of your left hand on the inner edge.

Move your right hand forward while moving your left hand backward.

Reverse the motion, and move your right hand backward while moving your left hand forward. Continue alternating back and forth for at least 15 seconds and up to a minute at a time on each foot.

The Toe Rotate Technique

This technique focuses all on your toes and offers greater flexibility, increased range of motion, and improved circulation in these digits.

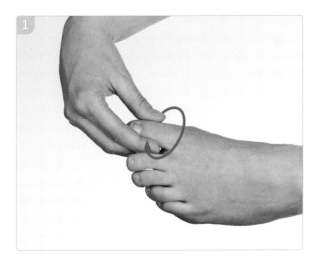

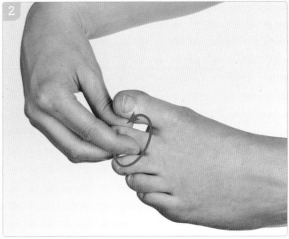

Keeping your foot steady with your left hand, gently grasp your big toe with the thumb and fingers of your right hand, and slowly move your toe in clockwise circles for 5 seconds and then reverse for counterclockwise circles for 5 seconds.

Keeping your foot steady with your left hand, gently grasp your second toe with the thumb and fingers of your right hand, and slowly move it in circles. Repeat for your remaining toes.

If you don't have a lot of movement in your ankles, feet, or toes, don't force any of these movements. Rather, start small with these two techniques. Many people experience progressively greater movement in their ankles, feet, and toes over time.

Relaxation Techniques for the Feet *(continued)*

These relaxation techniques are designed to compress and relax parts of your feet, to help improve the flow of blood and lymph in your feet.

The Fist Twist

The fist twist is designed primarily to help open capillary blood flow in your ball and pad, arch, and heel.

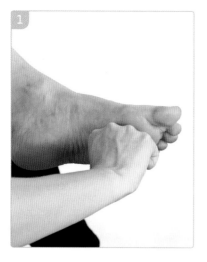

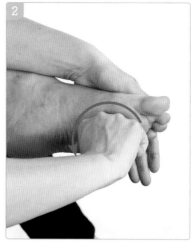

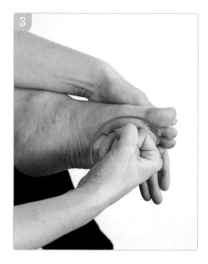

Make a fist with your right hand, and place it against the ball and pad of your left foot.

Hold the top of your foot with the palm of your left hand, and twist the fist of your right hand against your foot. Repeat several times.

Leave your left hand on top of your foot, move the fist of your right hand to the arch of your foot, and twist again. Repeat several times on your arch before moving on to your heel.

The Foot Sandwich

This technique increases circulation on the bottom of the foot, but primarily is designed to help with circulation on the top of the foot—an area that normally gets very little stimulation or movement throughout the day.

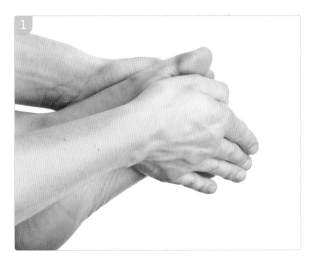

Place your left palm on top of your foot, near your toes, and place your right palm directly below it, on the bottom side surface of your foot. Squeeze your foot, and without rubbing over your skin, move your hands in slow alternating circles, stretching the skin on top of your foot. Repeat several times for each part of the top of your foot.

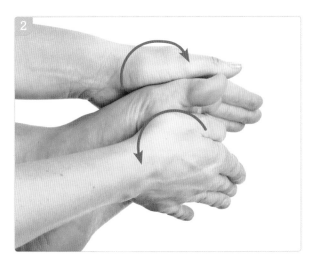

Move your hands halfway down your foot, and repeat. Move your hands again, near your ankle, and repeat.

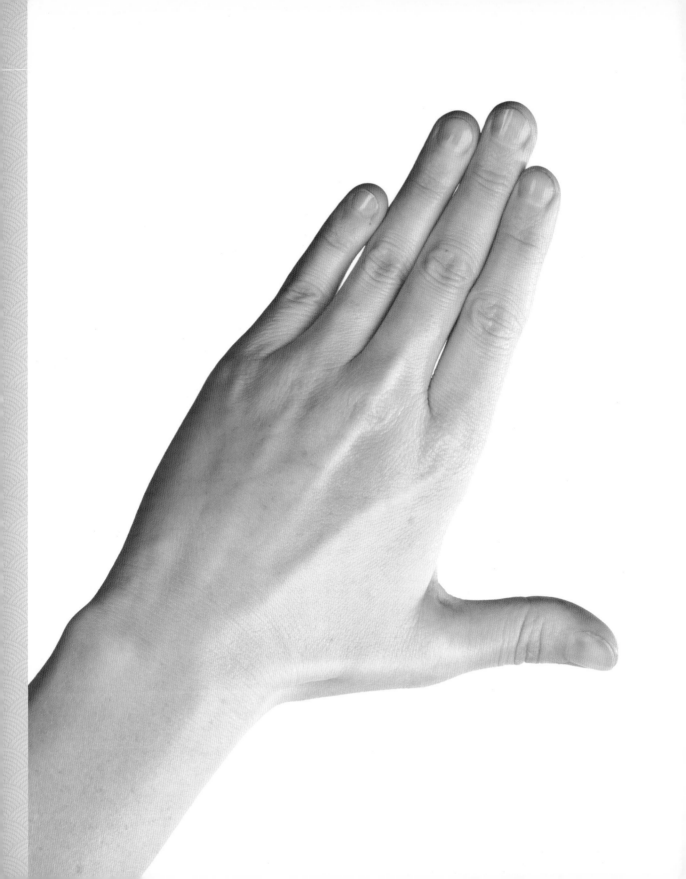

Part 5

Reflexology for the Hands

When reflexing the hands, many people have a tendency to work too deeply, especially on the palms, which can tax the hand doing the work. You don't want to strain your reflexing hand and thumb, and if your hand hurts, you probably won't work on hands for very long. Rather, work lighter for longer. Notice as you work that the tissue on your palm is softer close to the skin and the muscles closer to the bones are harder. Instead of pushing deep into the harder tissue, work across, between the soft surface tissue and hard deeper tissue. As you do this for a while, the firmer tissue will start to soften, allowing you to go deeper, with no more effort, strain, or discomfort on your working hand. In this part, I share an hour-long reflexology routine for your hands. Better health is literally at your fingertips!

The Thumb

Similar to your big toe, your thumb is home to reflexes that correspond to your head and neck. The longer you reflex your thumbs, the more your head and neck are likely to relax, which, in turn, will relax your chest and even your shoulders. When that happens, your breathing improves and your stress levels drop.

The tip of your thumb contains reflexes for the top of your head, the knuckle joint in the middle of your thumb is home to reflexes for the base of your head and the top of your neck, and the bottom of your thumb has reflexes that correspond to the bottom of your neck. Reflexing the big knuckle at the base of your thumb, where your thumb joins your hand, can be helpful for everything in the central part of your chest.

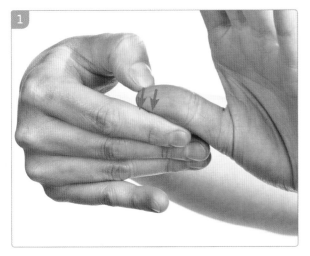

Place the pad of your right thumb on the thumb print surface of your left thumb. Thumb roll across your thumb, from the tip to the nearby joint.

As you work, don't expect the same degree of tenderness in your thumbs as you're likely to find in your big toes. Although most parts of your hands are less tender than your feet, your hands are still equally important to work on—not only on yourself, but also on others.

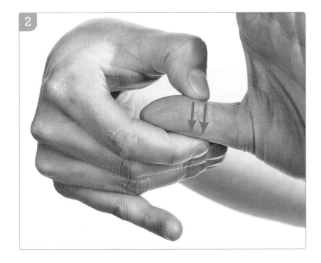

Repeatedly thumb roll across above, on, and below the knuckle joint.

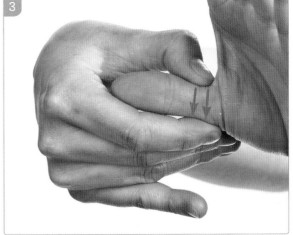

Thumb roll across the bottom half of your thumb, closest to your hand. Also spend some time thumb rolling across the big knuckle where your thumb joins your hand.

The Inner Edge of the Hand

Although there's just a short distance between the base of your thumb and your wrist, this inner edge of your hand is an important area to reflex, not only for the health of your spine, but also for everything inside your chest and abdomen.

This area holds reflexes for your uterus or prostate, urinary bladder, tail bone, sacrum, lumbar spine, and sciatic nerves in your wrist; your upper spine between your shoulder blades near the knuckle at the base of your thumb; and your middle spinal column in between.

Tension in your spine reduces nerve flow to organs, glands, and other structures in your chest and abdomen. The longer this reduced flow occurs, the greater the chance of diminished function of those organ, glands, and structures.

Frequently reflexing the inner edge of your hands helps reduce long-term tension, which allows for more optimal bioelectric flow to vital parts of your body for better health.

Notice the hard inner edge of the long bone between the base of your thumb and your wrist. On the palm side of that bone, feel a slight indentation or groove and the inner edge of the big muscle on the palm side of that bone. Reflex along all three—on the bone, in the groove, on the muscle.

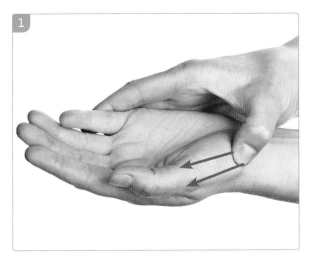

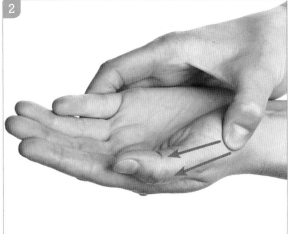

Rest the fingers of your right hand on the outer edge of your left hand, and place the pad of your right thumb at the base of the inner edge of your left hand, near your wrist. Thumb roll up toward your thumb.

Continue thumb rolling up the middle part of the inner edge of your hand.

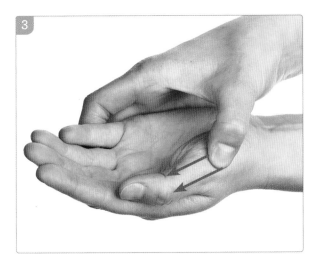

Thumb roll up the upper inner edge of your hand and just below the big knuckle at the base of your thumb.

The Palm

The palm of your hand is a relatively large area in terms of reflexology and contains numerous reflexes. It can help to think of this part of your hand in zones. Zone 1 covers the area between the base of your thumb down to your wrist. Zones 2 through 5 represent the heel of your hand, your palm, and the big knuckles where your fingers join your hand.

The area from the base of your thumb to your wrist is home to some of the largest and deepest muscles in your hand. Here you'll find reflexes for everything in the middle of your body—your spinal column, cord, and muscles, plus your central lymphatic and blood vessels. Reflexes for your chest are here, too, including your heart, trachea, esophagus, and thymus. Some lower abdomen reflexes are here as well, such as your uterus or prostate and urinary bladder. Closer to your wrist are reflexes for your lower abdominal area. For your chest near your sternum (breast bone), reflex closer to the base of your thumb.

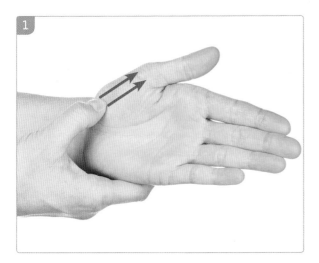

Rest the fingers of your right hand on the outer edge of your left hand, and place the pad of your right thumb at the base of your left hand, near your wrist. Thumb roll up toward your thumb.

If this part of your hand is tender or sore when you work on it, the discomfort might not be because of a problem in the midline of your body, but rather, just a sore muscle in your hand.

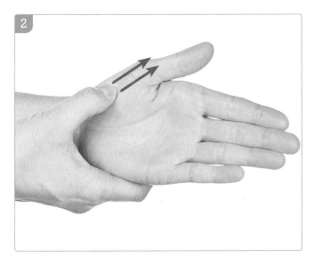

Continue thumb rolling up the middle part of your hand.

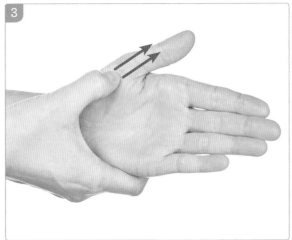

Thumb roll up to and over the big knuckle at the base of your thumb.

The Palm (continued)

Zones 2 through 5 represent the largest area on your palm and are home to reflexes for your lower abdominal pelvic area, your upper abdominal region, and your chest.

Reflexing your palm between the big knuckles below your index and middle fingers and the heel of your hand can be very helpful for relief of nausea, heartburn, and upset stomach. If you have stress or health issues anywhere in your chest, upper, mid, or lower abdomen, determine which zone or zones it's in, and reflex that zone as well as the adjacent zones. When you want to focus on a specific part, hold, or apply slow, small circles for a while.

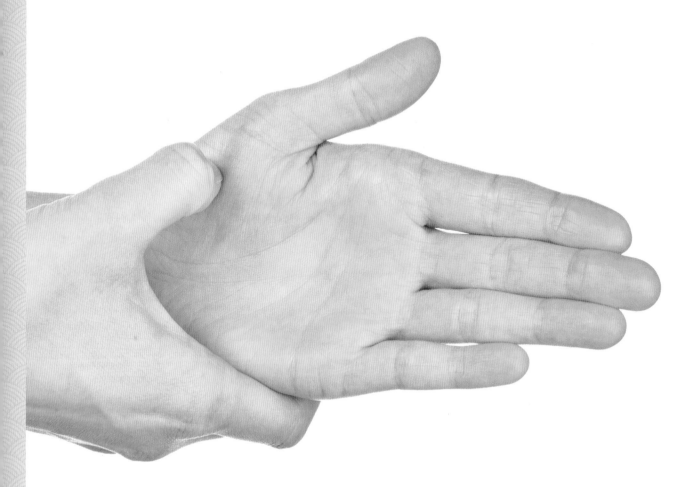

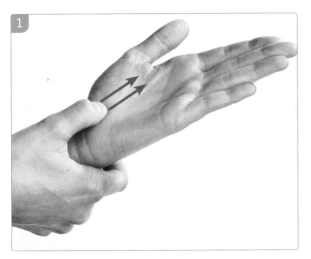

Rest the fingers of your right hand on the back of your hand, near your wrist, and place the pad of your right thumb near the palm side of your left wrist. Thumb roll up to the base of your left index finger.

Because some of the tissue on the palm side of your hand can be so deep, you might be tempted to reflex deeply with more pressure. It's better to start lightly, with a flatter thumb roll. As the tissue starts to soften, you can go deeper without straining your working hand or thumb. Also use a higher-angle thumb roll, reflexing more with the tip of your thumb. This helps you get into the deeper muscle layers closer to the bone.

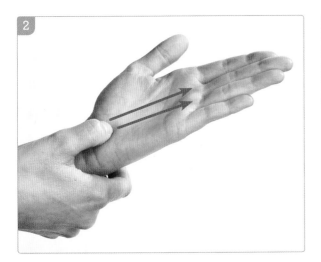

Repeat by thumb rolling from near your wrist up to the base of your fingers, overlapping a bit each time.

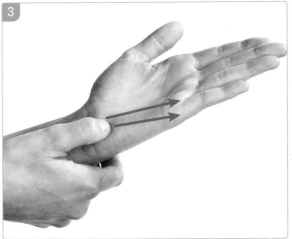

Thumb roll from your wrist, up to the base of your little finger.

The Big Web of the Hand

The big web of your hand sits between your thumb and the rest of your hand. If you stretch your thumb out to the side, you'll be better able to see your hand's big web.

The big web contains reflexes representing everything running parallel and next to your spine, from your collarbone down to your buttocks. Working in this area can be helpful for relaxing the long, ropelike the erector spinae muscles that run parallel to your spinal column.

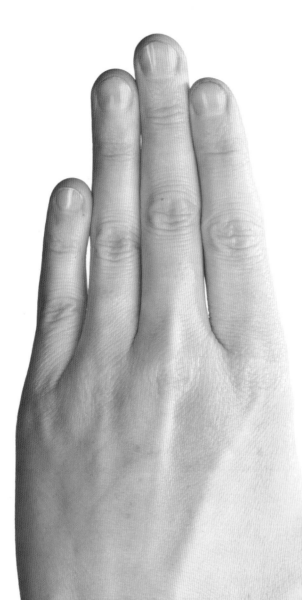

Running alongside where the big web connects to the long bone at the base of your index finger are some reflex points that aren't from reflexology maps, but rather from acupressure. The point called hoku, or large intestine 4, located in this intersection, is known to help with colon issues and also is beneficial for relief of headaches and sinus discomforts. Many people have found remarkable relief of headache and sinus problems by holding the hoku point for long periods of time. Avoid working your hoku if you're in your first trimester of pregnancy.

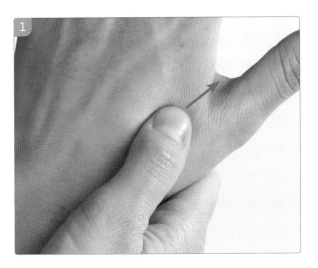

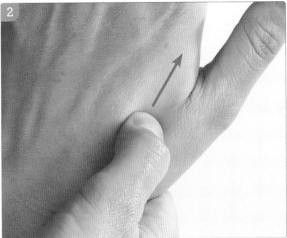

Starting near the bone at base of your thumb, squeeze your big web between tip of your index finger (on the palm side of your hand) and the tip of your thumb (on the back of your hand) with a high-angle thumb roll.

Thumb roll several times, reflexing the large, fleshy part of your big web, from near your wrist to the thinnest part of your big web.

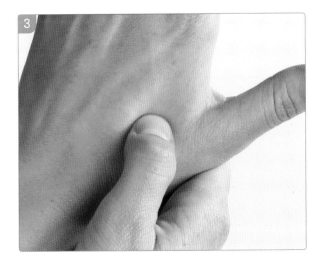

Move alongside the long bone below your index finger. Where you feel an area that's thicker, harder, or tenderer, stop and hold for 3 minutes on each hand for relief of normal headaches and up to 30 minutes on each hand for relief of migraines and sinus issues.

The Smaller Webs

Between your thumb and the rest of your hand is your big web. At the base of each of the rest of your fingers are smaller webs. These three smaller webs hold reflexes for your collarbone and your uppermost shoulder muscles.

Many people carry around tension in their shoulders. Some even live with frequent or ongoing discomfort where the base of their neck and the uppermost part of their shoulders connect. If you do, reflexing the three smaller webs of your hands can be quite helpful for reducing or eliminating upper shoulder pain and discomfort.

When you start to feel around on your smaller webs, you'll notice both thin tissue, near the edges of the webs, and thicker tissue just below that tissue, between the big knuckles at the base of your fingers where they join your hand. When reflexing your smaller webs, be sure to work both the thinner parts as well as the thicker parts.

You might find these webs to be quite tender. If so, reflex using lighter pressure for short periods of time every day or so.

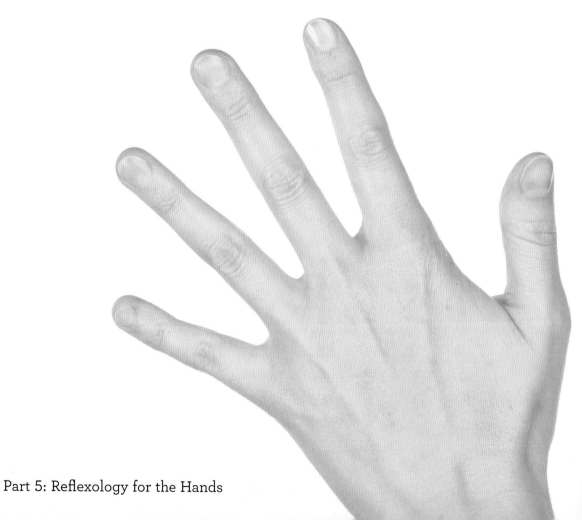

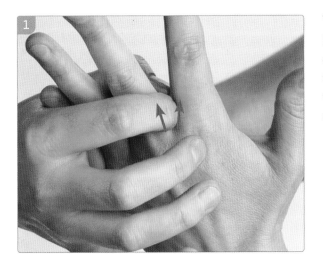

With your right hand, squeeze the small web between your index and middle fingers using the tip of your thumb (on the palm side of your hand) and the tip of your index finger (on the back side of the web). Then do a high thumb roll, pushing the web against the tip of your index finger with your thumb.

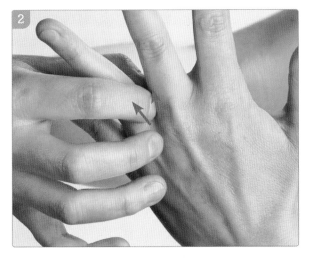

Move to the web between your middle finger and your ring finger, and repeat.

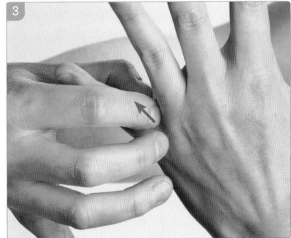

Move to the web between your ring finger and your little finger, and repeat.

The Outer Edge of the Hand

Because it's such a small area, the outer edge of your hand is often not given a lot of thought. However if you have hip, leg, arm, or elbow issues, you'll want to reflex this area between your wrist and the base of your little finger.

The outer edge of your hand holds reflexes for your foot, lower leg, knee, upper leg, hip, hand, wrist, and ovaries or testes (near your wrist); your upper arm and the muscles at the top of your arm (near the base of your fingers); plus your forearm and elbow (in between).

Your red blood cells and some of your white blood cells are made in your body's long and flat bones. The outer edge of your hand contains reflexes for most of the long bones in your arms and legs as well as for the flat bones of your hips. Anytime you have any short- or long-term issues related to your body's ability to produce either enough red blood cells or enough white blood cells, spend extra time reflexing the outer edge of your hand.

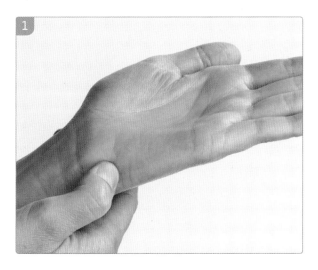

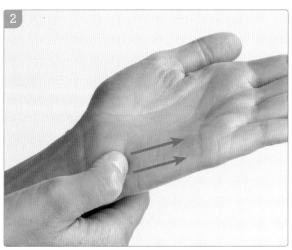

Rest the fingers of your right hand along the back of your left wrist, and place the corner of your right thumb on the outer edge of your left hand, near your wrist. Push in and out repeatedly until you find the spot that's the most tender, and hold.

Thumb roll over the entire area on the outer edge of your hand, near your wrist.

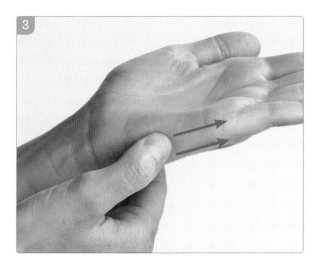

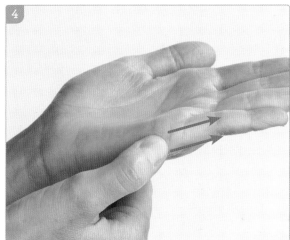

Move up a little higher along the outer edge of your hand, and continue to thumb roll to halfway up the outer edge of your hand, between base of your little finger and your wrist.

Keep thumb rolling up toward the rest of the outer edge of your hand until you reach the base of your little finger.

The Grooves on the Back of the Hand

If you have chest issues, especially breathing problems or shoulder issues (your shoulders are basically the back side of your chest), reflexing the grooves on the back of your hand often can be very helpful for relieving these and related discomforts.

The three grooves on the back of your hands contain reflexes for the front of your chest, including your chest muscles, breasts, ribs, and the muscles between your ribs; your inner chest, or your lungs and the lining of your lungs; and the back of your chest—the back of your ribs, your upper back muscles, and your shoulder muscles, shoulder blades, and the muscles between your shoulder blades.

Notice as you touch each groove that it contains three surfaces. What you're feeling are the bones on either side of the groove and the surface deep within each groove. Using a sideways index finger roll on all three surfaces, using the bony tip of your index finger as much as possible instead of the pad of your index finger, enables you to really get in the groove.

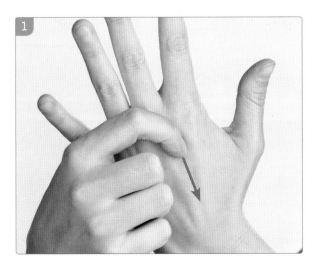

Rest the pad of your right thumb on the palm of your left hand, with the tip of your right index finger in the first groove at base of your second and third fingers. Sideways index finger roll two thirds of the way down toward your wrist.

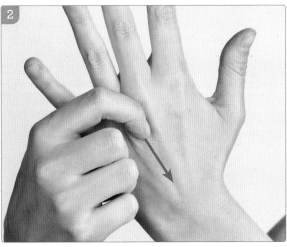

Continue holding with your thumb, but move your index finger to the next groove, and sideways index finger roll two thirds of the way down toward your wrist.

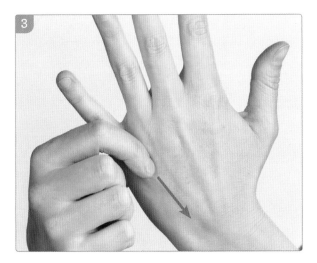

Repeat for the third groove, holding with your thumb, and sideways index finger rolling two thirds of the way down toward your wrist.

As you roll down each groove with the tip of your index finger, pay attention to where any tender spots might be in your hand. When you find these tender spots, don't stop reflexing them. Do work a little bit lighter, but continue to work on these tender spots for 5 to 10 minutes at a time every day or so.

Across the Back of the Hand

Reflexing the grooves on the back of your hand can be valuable for the front, inside, and back of your chest. Reflexing across the entire back of your hand several times, across the big knuckles where your fingers join your hand across the middle of your hand, and across the part of your hand closest to your wrist, benefits not only your chest, but also improves wellness in your upper abdomen and lower abdominal pelvic areas.

Mentally divide the back of your hand horizontally into three sections. The section closer to your big knuckles contains reflexes for your chest. The third closer to your wrist holds reflexes for your lower abdominal and pelvic musculoskeletal area. The third in between is for your upper abdominal area.

You might be tempted to do a three-finger roll on the back of your hand, using mainly the pads of your fingers. Although this will be valuable, you'll get better results by using a high finger roll, meaning rolling your three fingers so the bony tips of your fingers are doing most of the work. Using the bony tips help you do more detail work, for better results.

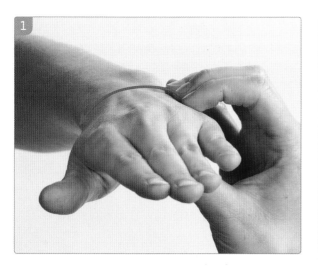

Rest the pad of the right thumb on your left palm, and place the pads of your right index, middle, and ring fingers on the outer edge of your left hand. Three-finger roll across the back of your big knuckles toward tips of your fingers.

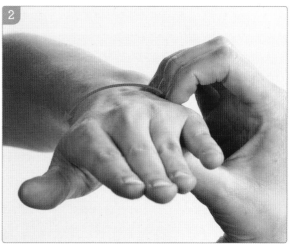

Move your three fingers down to the middle of the back of your hand, and three-finger roll across again.

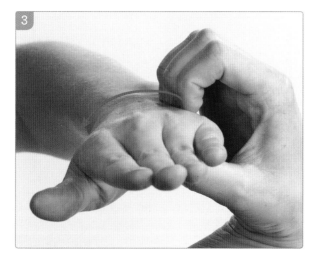

Move your three fingers down to the part of your hand closest to your wrist, and three-finger roll across again. Be sure to reflex across your wrist, too.

Across the Palm

Your palm, from the base of your fingers to your wrist, contains reflexes for everything from the top of your shoulders (or the top of your chest), to your internal and external upper abdomen, to your internal and external lower abdominal pelvic area. Reflexing across your palm offers benefits for all these areas.

You can reflex your palm at different times during a reflexology session. You could do work on it at the beginning of the routine or after working up the various zones of your palm.

However, if your thumb has been doing a lot of work during a session, it'll need a rest. While you're finger rolling the grooves on the back of your hand and working across the back of your hand, the muscles of your working hand, especially your thumb, can have a bit of a break so they don't become overworked or strained.

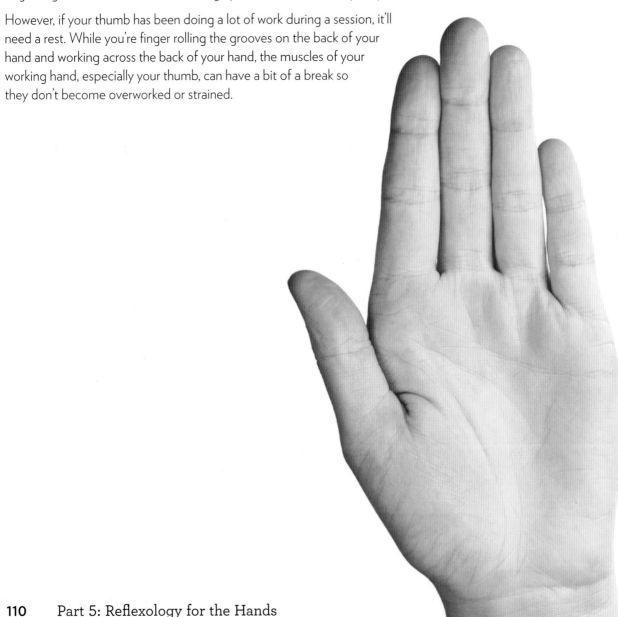

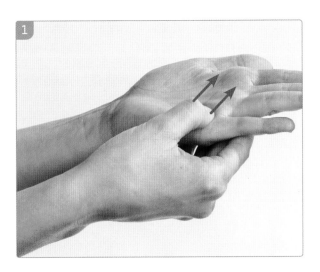

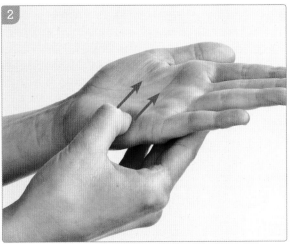

Rest your right fingers on the back of your left hand, and place the pad of your right thumb on your left palm, at the base of your little finger. Thumb roll across your big knuckles, overlapping a bit each time you work across.

Move your thumb down, and reflex across the soft part of your palm, again overlapping a bit as you go across.

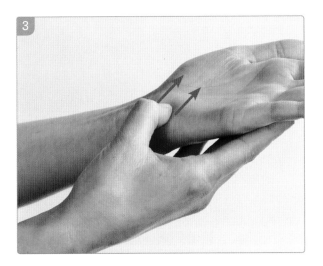

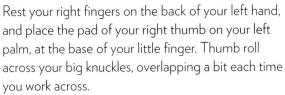

Move your thumb down to the heel of your hand, and reflex across. Be sure to reflex your wrist as well, again overlapping each time across.

The Three Soft Sides of the Fingers

You have two sets of reflexes for your head and neck—one set in your thumbs and the other in your fingers—so if you don't have much time, you can reflex your thumbs thoroughly. However, if you have extra time, it's worth it to reflex the soft sides of your index, middle, ring, and little fingers as well, for an additional benefit for your head and neck.

Think of your fingers as divided into three sections: the tip end between your end knuckle and your fingertip, the middle section between your two knuckles, and the base section between your lower knuckle and the big knuckle where your finger joins your hand. On each of these sections, you have a hard side, on the back of your finger, where your skin is close to your bone, and three soft sides. You'll reflex the soft sides of each section separately, starting with your little finger.

The tip end of your fingers contain reflexes for your head, the middle section has reflexes for your head and neck, and the base section is home to reflexes for your neck.

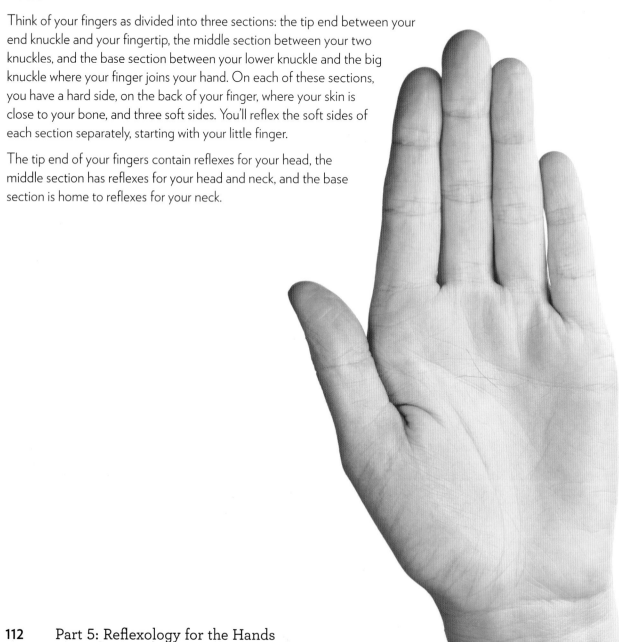

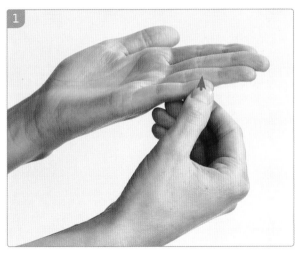

Cradling the tip end of your left little finger in your right index and middle fingertips, thumb roll the soft sides of the end section.

With three joints, your fingers can be very flexible. If your fingers are too flexible to reflex in the way described in the instructions, you can wrap the fingers of your right hand around each left finger as you thumb roll with your right thumb. This will make your finger more secure in your grip.

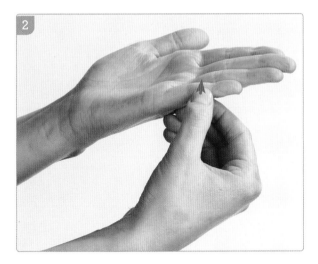

Move to the middle section of your little finger, and thumb roll the soft sides of the middle section.

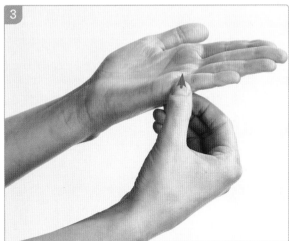

Move to the base section of your little finger, and thumb roll again.

Repeat with your ring, middle, and index fingers.

The Hard Sides of the Fingers and Thumb

Your fingers have three soft sides and one hard side, where your skin is closer to bone than soft tissue. Because the three softer sides are, well, softer, you can get a little more penetration into the tissue and feel like you're accomplishing more than when reflexing the hard, back side. But don't skip the back, hard surface of your fingers. This area is especially valuable to reflex.

Your fingers and your thumbs contain reflexes for everything in your head and neck. The bones near the tip end of your fingers and thumbs have reflexes for your head. The bone in the middle section of your fingers, between the knuckles, and section of your thumb between your knuckle and your thumbnail have reflexes for your head and neck. The section closest your big knuckles house reflexes for your neck.

Reflexing the back of your fingers and thumbs can be done with a thumb roll, but you can do more detail work with the bony tips of your fingers. If you like, you can start with a thumb roll and change to an index finger and middle finger roll.

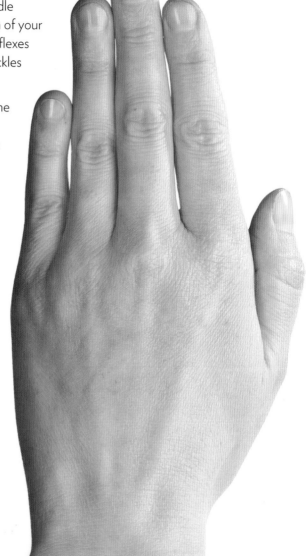

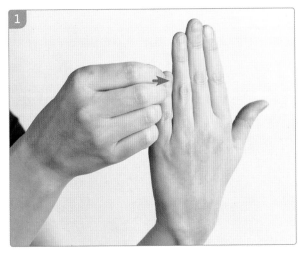

Reflexing the part of your thumb between the base of your thumbnail and your first knuckle can give great relief for dental pain as well as nose and facial injury discomfort. If you have any such issues, reflex this area for a longer time.

Place the pad of your right thumb against the palm side surface of your left little finger's tip end section. Place the pads of your right index and middle fingers on the hard side of this section. Index and middle finger roll end section, from the knuckle to the tip.

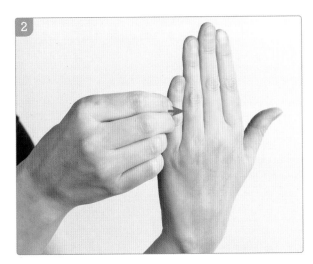

Move to the middle section of your little finger, and index and middle finger roll the middle section.

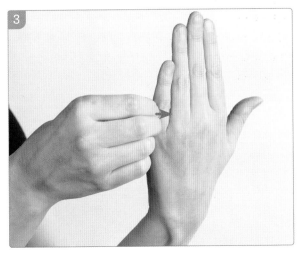

Move to the base section of your little finger, and index and middle finger roll again.

Repeat with your ring, middle, and index fingers and your thumb.

Relaxation Techniques for the Hands

These relaxation techniques are a perfect treat for your hands after they've performed a reflexology routine on your feet or ears (or your hands) and might be tired or sore. These techniques compress and relax various areas of your hand, which helps improve the flow of blood and lymph throughout this busy body part.

The Fist Twist

The fist twist is designed primarily to help open capillary blood flow in the big knuckles at the base of your fingers, the soft palm of your hand, and heel of your hand.

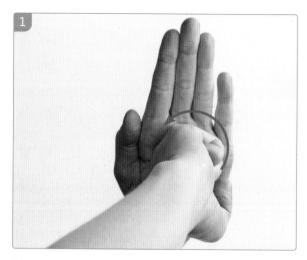

Place the fist of your right hand against the palm side surface of your left hand. Arrange it on the lower half of the your fingers, closet to your palm, as well as on the big knuckles at the base of your fingers, and twist your right hand.

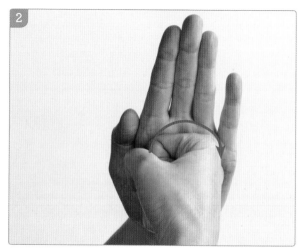

Lift your right hand, move it down a little, and repeat the fist twist on your palm and the heel of your hand.

The Finger Rotate

The finger rotate is designed to help improve circulation at the base of your fingers and in your big knuckles, where your fingers join your hands. It also can increase the range of motion in your fingers and thumbs.

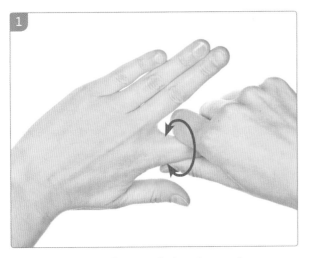

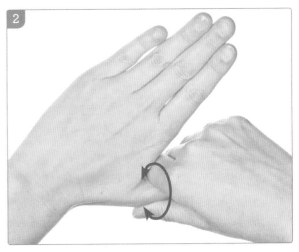

Wrap the fingers of your right hand around your left index finger, squeeze gently and stretch gently. Without letting go, rotate several times in one direction and then rotate several times in the other direction. Repeat on your middle, ring, and little fingers.

Wrap your right fingers around your left thumb, squeeze firmly and stretch gently. Without letting go, rotate several times in one direction and then rotate several times in the other direction.

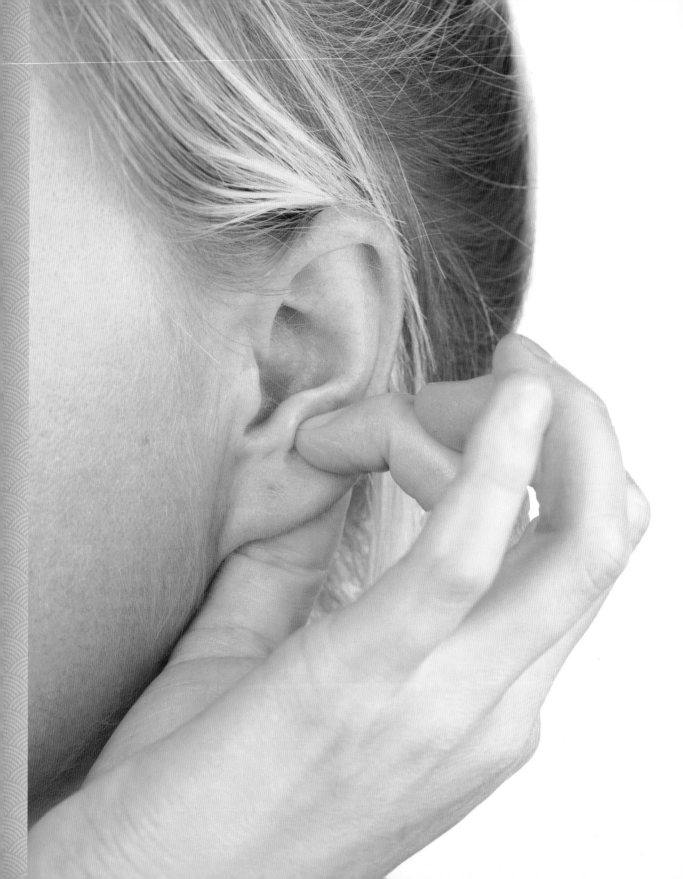

Reflexology for the Ears

Foot reflexology is quite well known, and hand reflexology is gaining in popularity. But you might not have heard much about ear reflexology until now.

We've known about a few isolated reflex points on the outer ear for centuries, but it was only in 1957 that a full reflex map was discovered on the ear, similar to those on the feet and hands. Like reflexology on those other areas, you can reflex, hold, and press areas on your outer ear to help your body restore and heal itself. In addition, one of the features that surprises many people—even those who practice other reflexology fairly regularly—is how relaxing the results of ear reflexology can be. In Part 6, you can try it for yourself as you learn how to work on all the parts of your outer ear using ear reflexology.

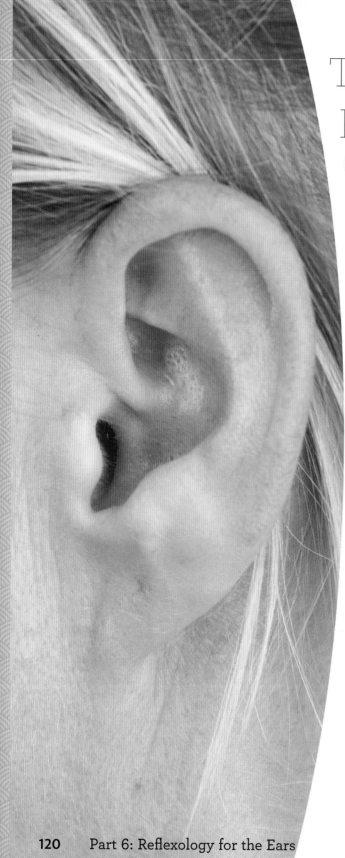

The Earlobe and Lobe Ridge

For such a small place, your earlobe contains numerous reflexes. It's home to reflexes for all the bones in your head, several specific parts of your brain, your eyes, your middle and inner ear, your teeth and gums, and your tonsils.

Your lobe ridge is located at the top of your earlobe. To find it, place your finger on the middle of your earlobe, halfway between your face and the back edge of your ear. Move your finger straight up to the hard cartilage—that's your lobe ridge. It contains more reflexes for parts of your head.

Very slowly flowing over your earlobe and lobe ridge and holding your brain reflexes not only helps with headaches, but also dramatically relaxes and reduces stress for your entire body—usually in under 2 minutes! It's best to do this with your elbows resting on a desk- or tabletop so you don't tire your shoulders.

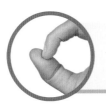

Use the tip of your index finger against the pad of your thumb with your earlobe in between.

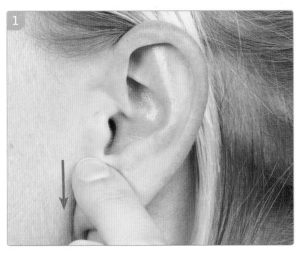

With the pad of your thumb behind your earlobe and the tip of your index finger in front, squeeze your earlobe at the top, where your lobe and your face connect. Very slowly flow down with your finger and thumb.

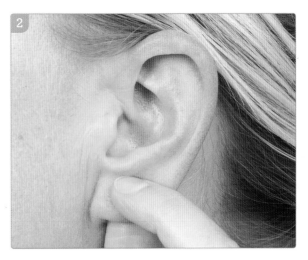

With the pad of your thumb behind and the tip of your index finger in front, squeeze the top of your earlobe. Slowly flow down the middle of your earlobe, and repeat down the back of your earlobe.

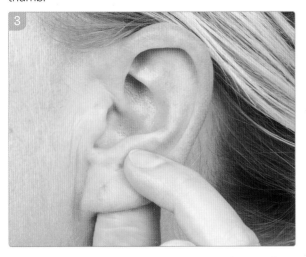

With the pad of your thumb behind and the tip of your index finger in front, squeeze and hold the area between your earlobe and your lobe ridge.

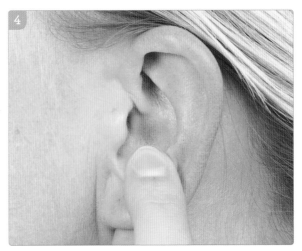

With the pad of your thumb behind and the tip of your index finger in front, firmly squeeze and hold your lobe ridge.

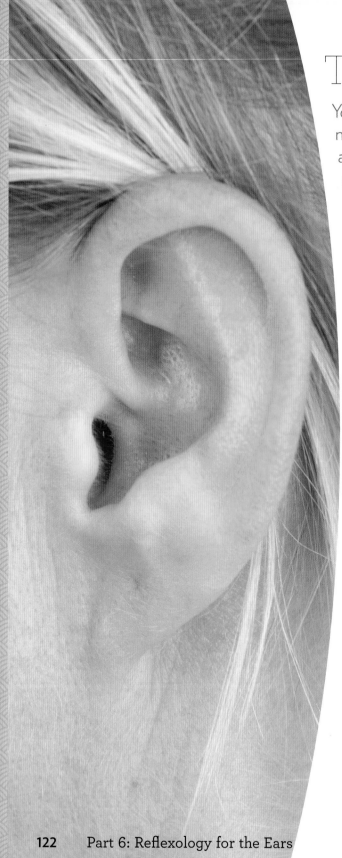

The Middle Ridge

Your ear's middle ridge has reflexes for your neck, middle spine, breasts, ribs, external abdominal muscles, and your thyroid and parathyroid glands.

Reflexing the lower 1 inch (2.5cm) of your ear's middle ridge can bring dramatic pain relief and increased range of motion to your neck. The longer you hold the neck reflex, the more benefit you'll receive. So many people carry around tension in their neck, it would be wise for just about everybody to work on their neck reflexes at least a few times a week.

Your neck muscles are connected into your head, chest, and shoulders, so the more your neck relaxes, the more your head, brain, sinuses, shoulders, chest muscles, and lungs will relax, too.

When holding reflex points or areas on your ear, use enough pressure to still be comfortable on your ear and at the same time not strain your fingers, thumbs, or hands.

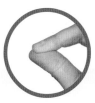

Unless otherwise instructed, use the pad of your index finger against the pad of your thumb with your ear in between.

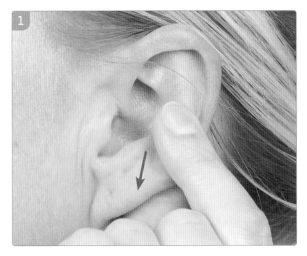

Place the pad of your thumb behind the entire length of your middle ridge and the pad of your index finger on the front side. Slowly flow with your index finger, keeping your thumb stationary.

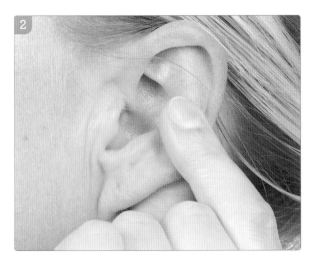

With the pad of your thumb behind the lower 1 inch (2.5cm) of your middle ridge and the pad of your index finger on the front, squeeze and hold.

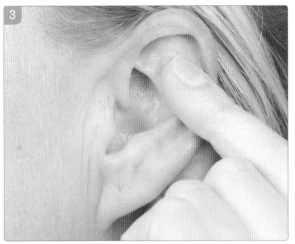

With the pad of your thumb behind the wider part of your middle ridge and the tip of your index finger on the front, squeeze and hold.

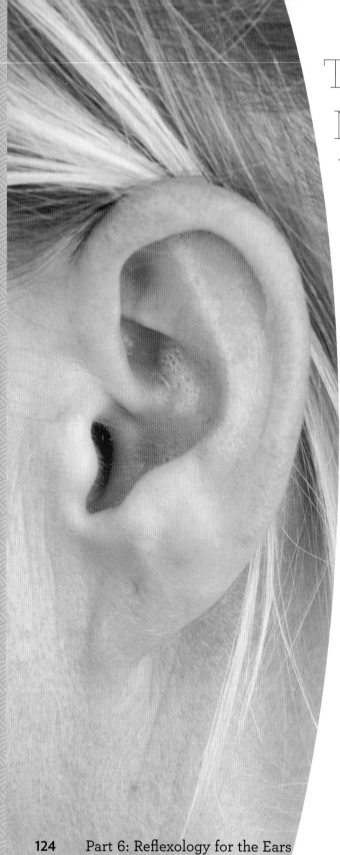

The Wide and Narrow Ridges

Your ear's wide ridge holds reflexes for your upper leg, knee, lower leg, ankle, heel, foot, and toes. Your narrow ridge holds reflexes for your lower back bones (lumbar, sacrum, tailbone), hips, and sciatica. It also has a master point called the *sympathetic point,* for circulatory issues in your body.

Reflexing the heel, foot, and toe reflexes on your ear's wide ridge can help with heel spurs, foot discomforts, and injured or stubbed toes.

Reflexing your narrow ridge has been known to be remarkably helpful for relieving pain and discomfort related to the lower back, hips, and sciatica. Holding your narrow ridge for anywhere between 10 to 20 minutes or more at a time has proven to yield dramatic results in many cases. To avoid taxing your arms and shoulders during this time, be sure your elbows are comfortably resting on a desk- or tabletop when reflexing your narrow ridge.

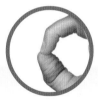

Using the tip of your index finger against the tip of your thumb with your earlobe in between helps you target a specific area.

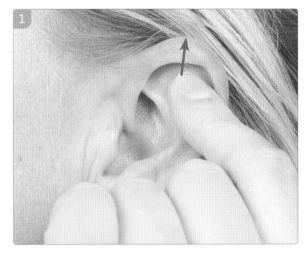

Place the pad of your thumb behind your wide ridge and the tip of your index finger on front side. Flow slowly upward, toward the top of your ear, several times, overlapping each time.

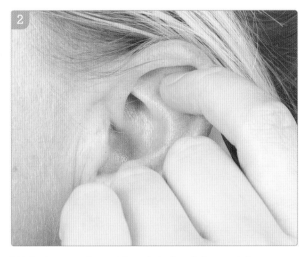

With the tip of your thumb behind the middle part of your wide ridge and the tip of your index finger on front side of your knee reflex, hold.

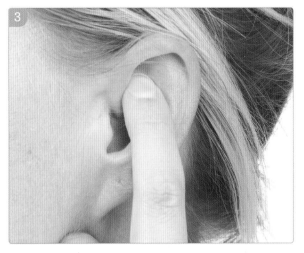

Place tip of your index finger underneath your narrow ridge. While pushing upward gently, flatten your narrow ridge by pushing it against your head.

The Wide and Narrow Ridges   **125**

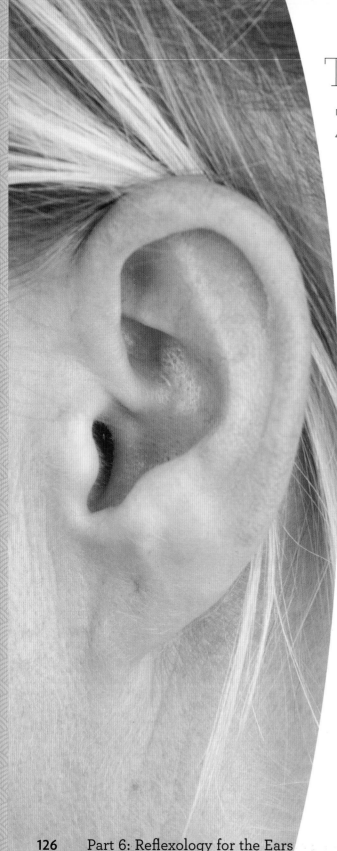

The Divine Gate, Zero Point, and Master Endocrine Point

The *divine gate*, also called *shen men*, is the most widely known reflex point on the ears. It has broad applications for the health of your entire body. It's useful for overall homeostasis and pain relief anywhere in the body, as well as for antidepression and chemical dependency issues.

The *zero point* is equivalent to the solar plexus in the upper abdomen. As you reflex this point, you can help relax your lower chest, your diaphragm, and your upper and lower abdomen.

The *master endocrine point* is home to the pituitary gland reflex. Your pituitary gland, when functioning properly, releases chemicals that help the other endocrine glands throughout your body produce and release their chemicals and hormones more efficiently.

The best way to reflex these areas is to simply hold them. The longer you hold, the greater the results you're likely to experience.

The divine gate, zero point, and master endocrine point are a category of reflex points on the ears called master points. Each has broad impact on other parts or functions of your body.

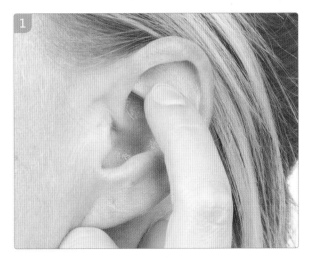

Place the tip of your index finger on the front of the narrowest part of your triangular valley (your divine gate), and hold.

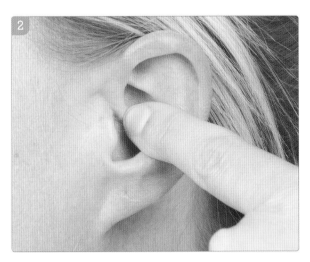

Place the tip of your index finger firmly against the notch between the root of your outer ridge and your inner ridge (your zero point), and hold.

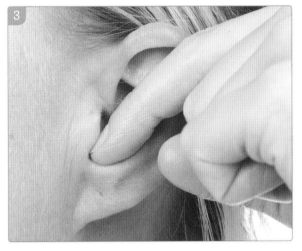

Place the tip of your index finger or your thumb on your notch ridge (your master endocrine point), and hold.

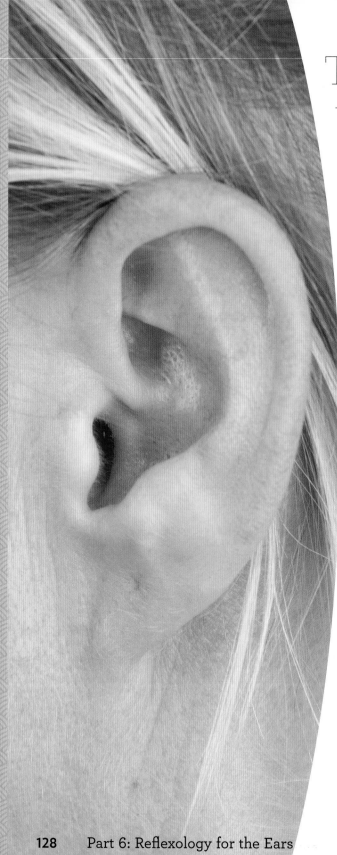

The Lower and Upper Valleys, Inner Ridge, and Triangular Valley

It can be amazing to think about how many reflex points and areas cover your ears—so many in such a small space!

Your ear's lower valley contains reflexes for your heart, lungs, trachea, mouth, throat, esophagus, muscular point, and subcortex. Your inner ridge has reflexes for your stomach, liver, and spleen. Your upper valley is home to reflexes for the small and large intestine, ileocecal valve, gallbladder, pancreas, kidney, ureter, urinary bladder, and prostate. And your triangular valley holds reflexes for the uterus, leg, histamine point, asthma point, hepatitis point, and constipation point.

While slowly and firmly flowing over these areas, notice the slight differences in textures, on and slightly under the surfaces of your ear. Also notice when you flow over a tender spot. When you find texture irregularities or tender spots, stop and hold these areas. These frequently can be an indication of a current or past imbalance (a trauma or an injury) in the related part of your body.

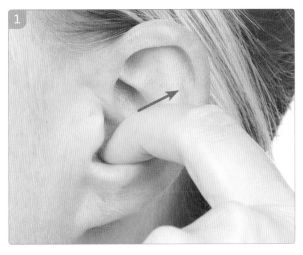

Place the tip of your index finger in your lower valley against your head, near your ear canal. Slowly flow back repeatedly until you cover the entire surface.

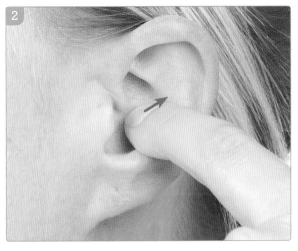

Place the tip of your index finger on your inner ridge and move back slowly, stopping to hold either your stomach, liver, or spleen reflex.

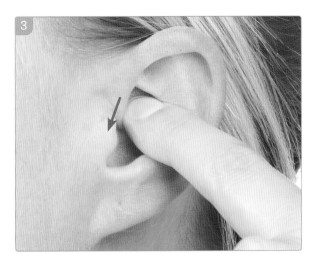

Place the tip of your index finger in your upper valley, against your head, near your inner ridge. Slowly flow forward repeatedly until you cover the entire surface.

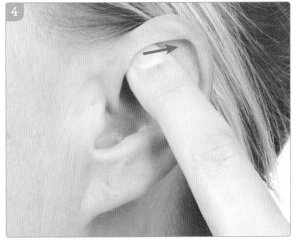

Place the tip of your index finger in your triangular valley and flow slowly but firmly until the entire area is covered.

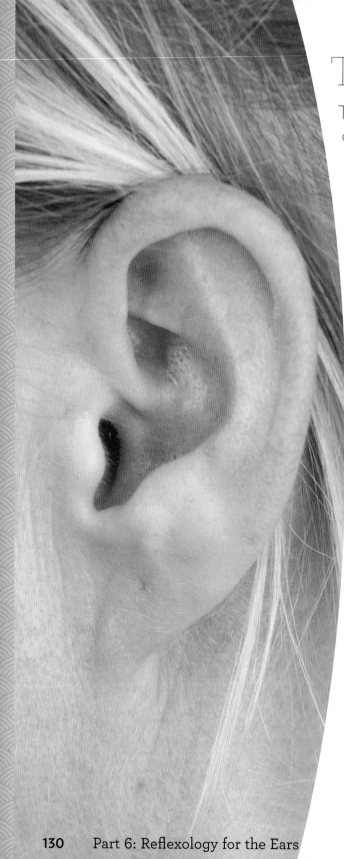

The Outer Valley

The indentation at the bottom of your ear's outer valley is home to your jaw reflex. Moving upward from there are reflexes for your shoulder, upper arm, elbow, forearm, wrist, hand, and fingers.

While holding your jaw reflex, or your TMJ point, for relief of pain and discomfort in your jaw, move the tip of your thumb and index finger very slowly in alternating circles. Be sure you're not rubbing over your skin but instead moving your skin over the underlying tissue.

Reflexing your shoulder reflexes in your ear's outer valley can be extremely powerful for relieving any type of discomfort associated with this joint.

For even greater results, place the pad of your thumb across the back of your ear and the pad of your index finger on the front of your ear, on your neck and shoulder reflexes, and hold firmly. Usually within 3 or 4 minutes, you'll start to feel relaxation in your shoulder area. The longer you hold these two reflexes, the more relaxation you'll feel. Remember to rest your elbows on a desk- or tabletop while holding these reflexes.

Your elbow reflex is also a sleep disorders point, and your wrist reflex doubles as a skin disorders point.

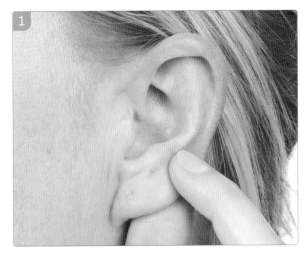

Place the tip of your index finger in the front indentation at the base of your outer valley and the tip of your thumb in the back. Squeeze and hold.

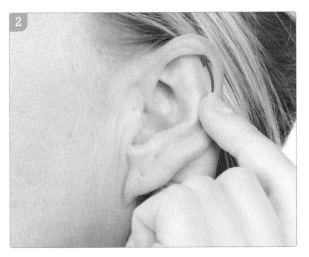

With the pad of your thumb behind your outer valley, and the tip of your index finger on the front side of your outer valley, slowly and firmly flow upward with your index finger.

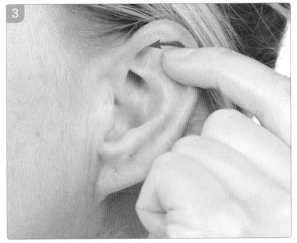

Moving the pad of your thumb higher behind the uppermost part of your outer valley, continue slowly and firmly flowing upward with the tip of your index finger.

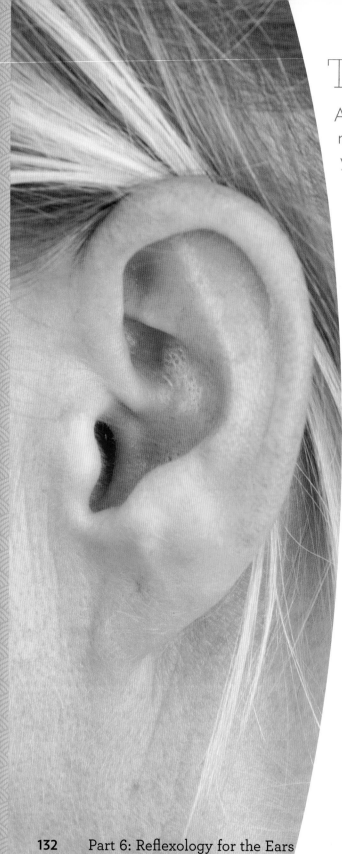

The Outer Ridge

Although it's long and thin, your ear's outer ridge is home to many reflexes. It contains your diaphragm and external genitalia reflexes (near your face); the allergy point (at the top of the arch); and your lower, middle, and upper spinal cord reflexes (from the bump down to your earlobe).

Your outer ridge also has three tonsil reflexes. Because it contains three tonsil reflexes as well as your spinal cord reflex, the outer ridge is said to be helpful for neuroendocrine conditions in the body.

The allergy point, located at the very top arch of your ear, can be helpful for reducing and eliminating allergic symptoms like those associated with food allergies and intolerances as well as respiratory reactions, such as for pollens and grasses in the air, and reactions to cat hair and dander, to mention a few.

As you're reflexing your outer ridge, you might find it easier to have your thumb behind your outer ridge and let your index finger do the reflexing work on the front side. At other times, it might be more effective to do the opposite, with your index finger behind your outer ridge and the tip of your thumb doing the work on the front side.

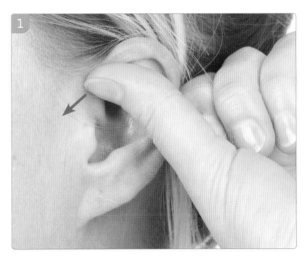

Place tip of your thumb at the root of your outer ridge and push firmly. Slowly flow forward toward your face and then upward toward the top of your outer ridge.

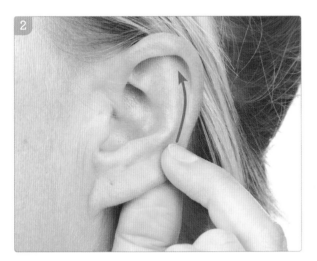

With the pad of your thumb behind your outer ridge, place the tip of your index finger in front, at the base, near your earlobe. Squeeze firmly and slowly flow upward toward the top of your outer ridge.

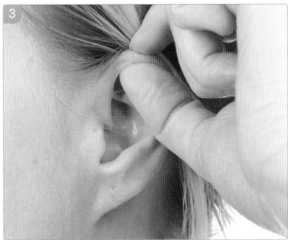

Place the tip of your thumb underneath the highest part of your outer ridge, and place the tip of your index finger on top of that ridge. Squeeze firmly and hold.

Relaxation Technique for the Ears

Because they're smaller than your feet or hands, and because they contain so many reflexes in such a compact space, your ears can really use a nice relaxing finish to a reflexology session.

This simple relaxation technique is a lovely way to end your time spent working on your ears. It's designed to provide a warm, soothing feeling, made by rubbing your hands together, getting you palms warm, and carefully cupping them over the ears without flattening them against the ears.

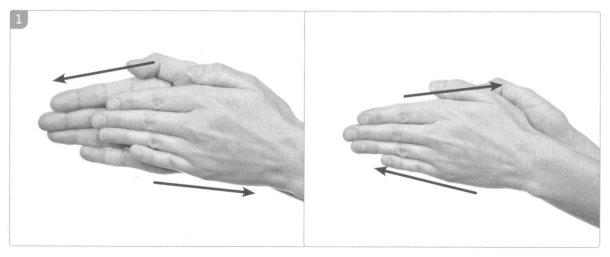

Place the palms of your hands together firmly, and rub them together, back and forth, very quickly until they start to feel warm.

In addition to feeling soothing for tired ears, there's an additional purpose to this relaxation technique. As the heat from your hands penetrates deep into the tissue of your outer ear, blood circulation and lymphatic flow increase, which helps capillaries be more open and able to take away chemicals you've broken down around the reflexes.

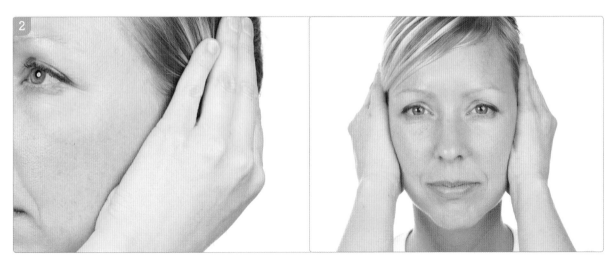

Very quickly cup your hands over your ears, being careful to not smash your ears or flatten them ears against your head. Hold for 10 to 15 seconds, and slowly bring your hands away from your ears before repeating a second time.

Your hands will likely become warmer the second time you do this; the third time, your hands should become *hot*. For these subsequent times, leave your hands cupped over but not touching your ears for up to 60 seconds. When you take away your hands, do it very slowly.

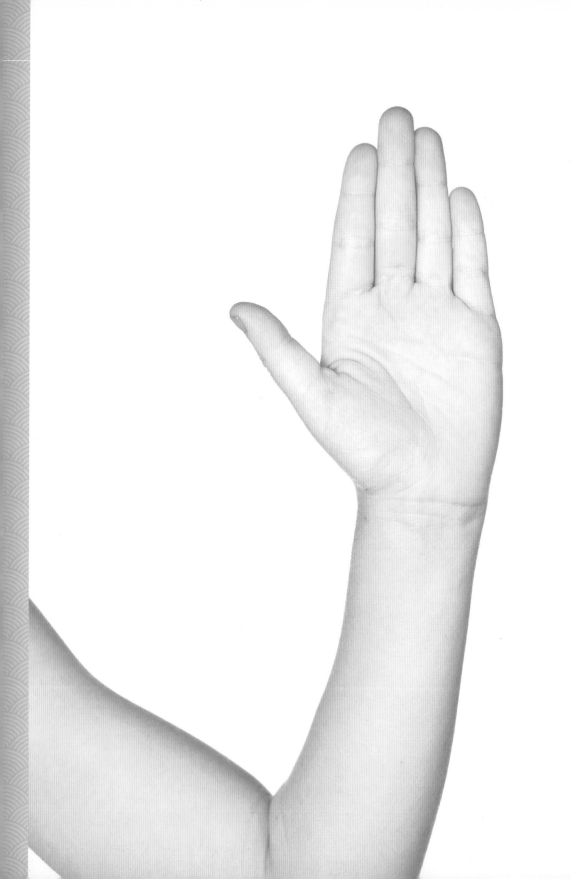

Part 7

Reflexology for Everyone

Reflexology is indeed for everyone, from babies and children, to adults and seniors. Whether you're looking to learn about reflexology that's specialized for you, as a woman or as a senior citizen, or you're seeking relief for your colicky baby or child with an ear infection, you've come to the right part.

In Part 7, you learn how women can use reflexology to relieve morning sickness or calm the symptoms of menopause. Parents can learn how to soothe a teething baby or quiet a fussy child. Even seniors can find beneficial reflexology in these pages, from help with circulation to relief from insomnia.

Reflexology for Women

Women experience a range of changes in hormonal activity, throughout all stages of life, from puberty through menopause. For women who become pregnant, the 9 months of pregnancy; labor and childbirth; the potential demands of breast-feeding; little or poor sleep; and the constant care newborns require place even greater physical and emotional demands on the gender. The result of these hormonal fluctuations can include menstrual cramps, yeast infections, ovarian cysts, menopause, hot flashes, and more, such as morning sickness during pregnancy.

Myriad chemical changes occur in a woman's body during her child-bearing years, an imbalance of which can manifest as more than a hundred different symptoms. You have several options for how to use reflexology for relief and prevention of these symptoms. You can target specific conditions, such as the stomach reflexes for nausea and morning sickness or the uterine reflexes for menstrual cramps.

Or you can reflex for the many different parts of the body involved in the chemical changes. For example, you reflex for the pineal gland, which triggers the part of the brain called the hypothalamus, which triggers the pituitary, which releases chemicals that affect the thyroid gland (temperature control of the body), and the adrenal glands (testosterone and other chemicals), the ovaries, and the uterus.

Chances are, you're not a trained reflexologist, so rather than try to remember all those specific reflex locations on the feet, hands, and ears, simply reflex the bottom of your big toes, the bottom of your feet, and the inner edge of your foot near your ankle. On your hands, work on your thumb, the palm of your hand, and the inner edge of your hand near your wrist. On your ears, reflex your earlobe and your lower, upper, and triangular valleys. This relaxing and rejuvenating routine covers all the necessary reflexes plus some other helpful areas as well.

Avoid working on the uterine reflexes in your feet, hands, and ears during the first trimester of pregnancy. Some believe it's okay to reflex these areas during the first three months of pregnancy, as long as you use only light pressure and do so for short periods of time, but when in doubt, it's best to err on the side of caution and avoid these reflexes during this time.

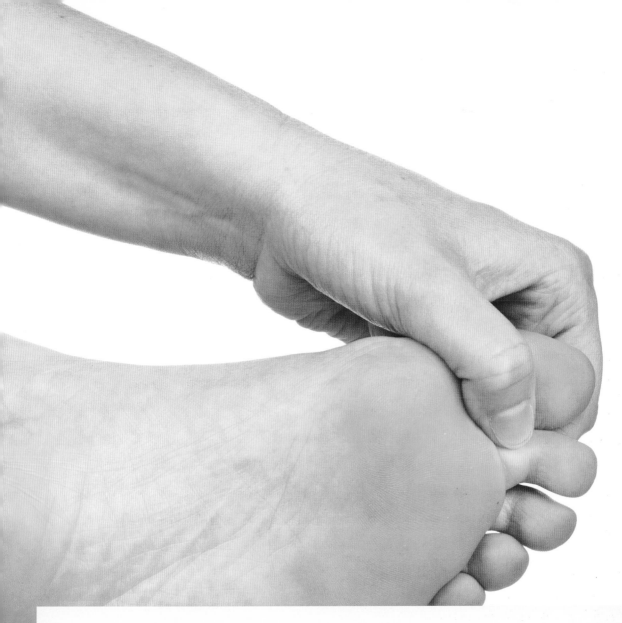

The first reflexology research study published in scientific literature was a 6-month study devoted to women and addressed 30 symptoms of premenstrual syndrome (PMS). Conducted at the American Academy of Reflexology (AAR), by Terry Oleson PhD, a number of AAR graduates, and me, "Randomized Controlled Study of Premenstrual Symptoms Treated with Ear, Hand, and Foot Reflexology" was published in *Obstetrics and Gynecology* in December 1993. Of the 30 PMS-related symptoms tracked every day during those 6 months, 15 were physical and 15 were psychological. The control group that did not receive reflexology during the 6 months showed no change in their symptoms, the placebo group reported a 19 percent reduction of their symptoms, and the group that received reflexology showed a 47 percent reduction of symptoms.

PMS and Menstrual Cramps

For relief of premenstrual syndrome (PMS) symptoms, especially cramps, work your uterine reflex. Sometimes, the uterine reflex in the triangular valley in your ear provides the quickest relief, but the uterine reflex in your feet is more consistent. Experiment to see which is best for you.

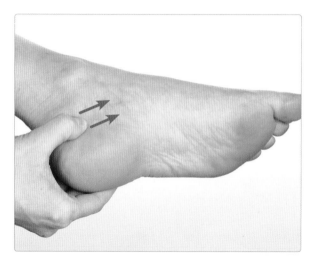

Work the inner edge of your foot, below your ankle.

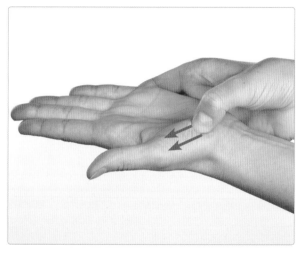

Reflex the inner edge of your hand, near your wrist.

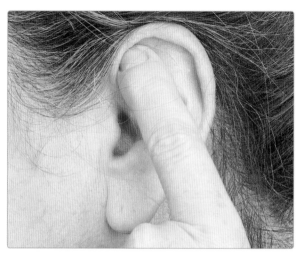

Hold the uterine reflex in triangular valley of your ear.

Yeast Infection Discomfort

Sometimes the uterine reflex in the ear's triangular valley provides the quickest relief for the symptoms of yeast infections, but the uterine reflex in the feet is more consistent. Try both to see which works best for you.

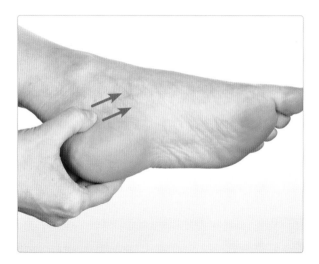

Work the inner edge of your foot, below your ankle.

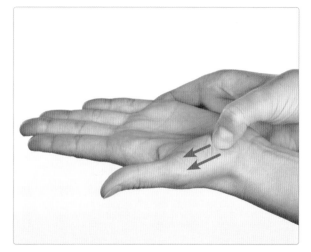

Reflex the uterine reflex on the inner edge of your hand, near your wrist.

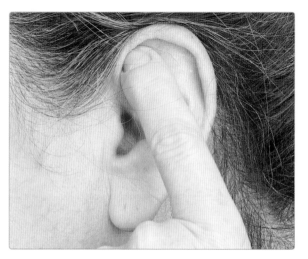

Hold the uterine reflex in your ear's triangular valley.

Ovarian Cyst

If you have pelvic pain or discomfort, an ovarian cyst might be the cause. (Check with your primary care physician.) To relieve some of the discomfort, index finger roll on the area below your outer ankle, progress to your hands, and hold the ovary reflex in your ear.

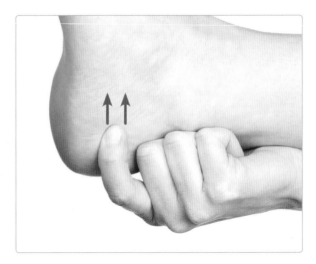

Index finger roll on the outer edge of your foot, below your ankle bone.

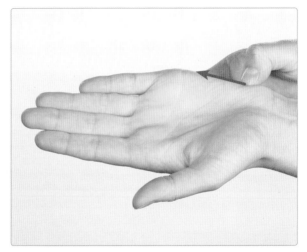

Also reflex the outer edge of your hand, near your wrist.

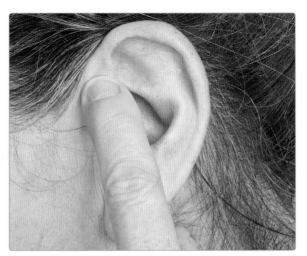

On your ear, hold the ovary reflex located on the outer ridge.

Morning Sickness

Morning sickness is a common ailment for women in their first trimester of pregnancy. For relief, work on the arch on your foot and all over the soft palm of your hand. Both areas are equally effective for relief. Then, on your ears, hold the stomach reflex.

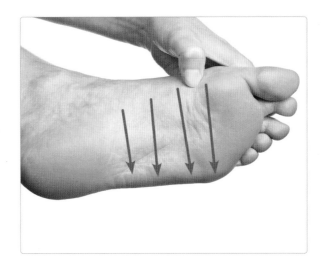

Reflex your entire arch.

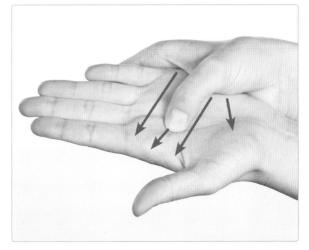

Work on the full area of your palm.

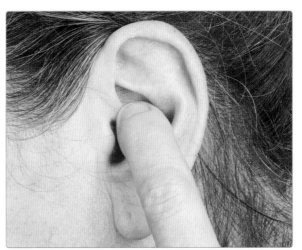

Hold the stomach reflex on the middle ridge of your ear.

Menopause

For relief of the numerous and varying symptoms of menopause, work on your uterine reflexes. Spend a lot of time working on the uterine reflex on your feet, and repeat several times a day.

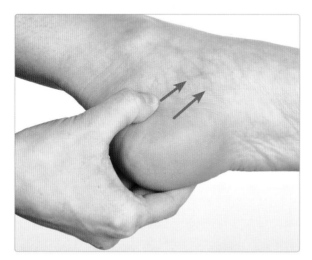

Reflex the uterine reflex and along the inner edge of your foot, below your ankle.

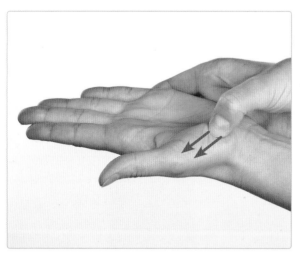

Apply gentle pressure along the inner ridge of your hand, near your wrist.

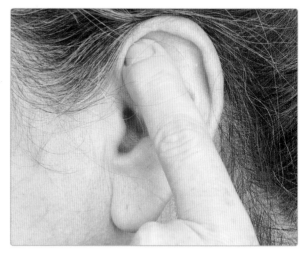

Work on the uterine reflex in the triangular valley.

Hot Flashes

To alleviate the discomfort of the hot flashes, work the uterine reflexes on your feet and hands. Then, hold the tip of your index finger gently on your endocrine point, in your ear's notch ridge.

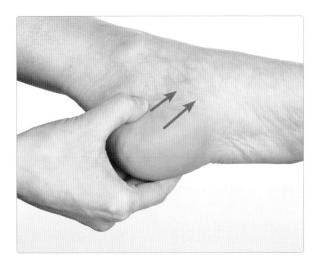

Work all along the inner edge of your foot, below your ankle.

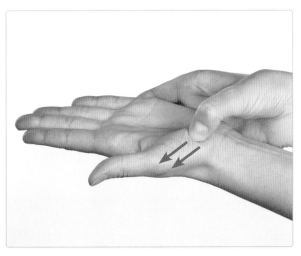

Reflex the inner edge of your hand, near your wrist.

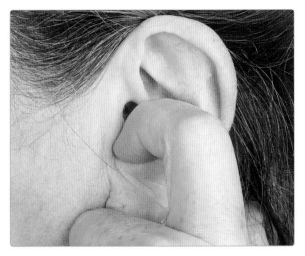

Apply gentle pressure to and hold your endocrine point.

Reflexology for Babies and Children

Have you ever noticed that young children often suck their thumb on one hand while holding their earlobe with the other hand? Isn't it interesting that both their thumbs and their earlobes have reflexes for the head and brain? Is it possible—of course, without really realizing it—they're soothing, relaxing, and comforting themselves by reflexing their brain reflexes?

I had just gotten to my friend's house when she asked me to work on Ben, her 6-year-old son. About an hour earlier, he had been climbing on a jungle gym, fell a several feet, and landed on concrete, face first. The skin on his face wasn't broken, but his nose hurt and there was no sign of his usual high energy. I moved him to a reclining chair, and with the soft pad of my index finger, worked on his nose and face reflexes on one of his big toes, between the base of the nail and the knuckle closest to the nail.

After about 3 minutes of reflexology, Ben began to get a slightly restless—an encouraging sign. When I worked on the same part of his other big toe, he settled down again. It was about another 3 minutes until he again became a little bit restless. This pattern continued for another couple cycles with each of his big toes. Within 15 minutes of starting, he was sitting up and looking around—another good sign. His pain was gone, the color had returned to his face, and his energy level was rapidly increasing.

Youngsters are very sensitive and can recover fairly quickly—a good thing since they usually can't stay still for much longer than 5 minutes. Ben's case, however, was extreme because his fall had not only hurt his nose, but had also given his head and brain quite a jolt.

While visiting another friend, her 6-month-old baby started crying and fussing. She tried to comfort her daughter, but the baby kept fussing. I suggested she put pads of her thumbs on the bottom of her baby's feet and hold gently. Within a minute, the baby had stopped fussing, and within 2 minutes, she had fallen asleep.

The purpose of these stories is to show how easily you can help babies and children with foot, hand, and ear reflexology. The key is to work for short periods of time—5 to 10 minutes max for those under 5—and to do so *very lightly*.

Colic, teething, fussiness, and ear infections are common for babies and little children. With reflexology, you can help them with these and other issues.

> Babies and children grow at such a rapid rate that their bodies and chemistry changes almost by the day. A little reflexology each week can go a long way toward helping make their journey through those years more comfortable and physically and emotionally balanced.

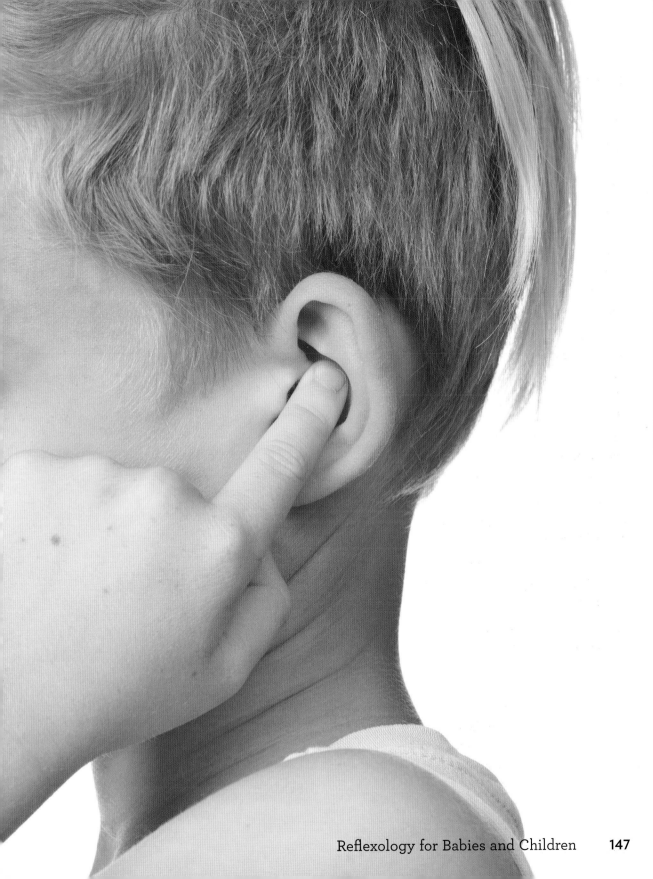

Colic

When working on babies and children, especially colicky babies, apply light pressure using the pads of your thumbs and fingers instead of the tips. Gently hold the reflexes just for a few minutes at a time.

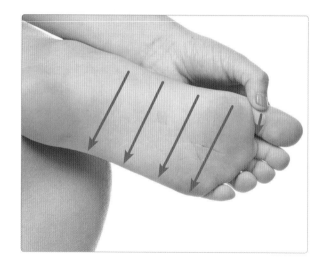

Gently work the base of the big toe, the ball of the foot, the pad, and the arch.

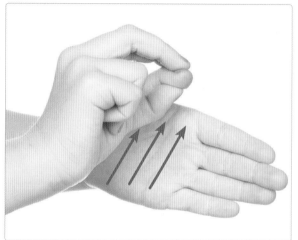

Lightly reflex the thumb, all of the palm, and the heel of the hand.

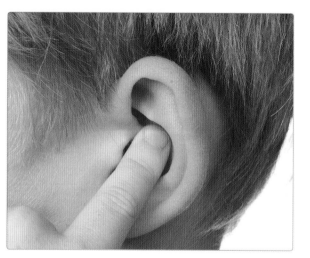

Softly hold the zero point on the ear.

Teething

When reflexing teething babies' feet, hands, and ears, do so very lightly. Work across the area between the bottom of the nail and the nearby knuckles of the big toe and thumb.

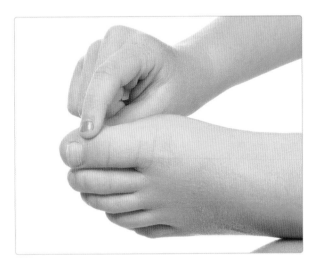

Gently reflex across the top of the big toe, between the bottom of the toenail and the middle knuckle.

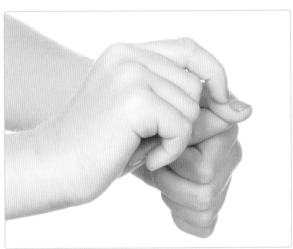

Work across the back of the thumb, between the bottom of the fingernail and the middle knuckle.

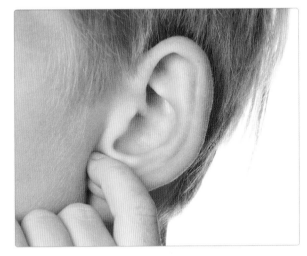

Gently hold the upper earlobe, near the face.

Fussiness

When working on fussy little ones, use the entire pad of your thumb, between the tip and the knuckle, and hold gently.

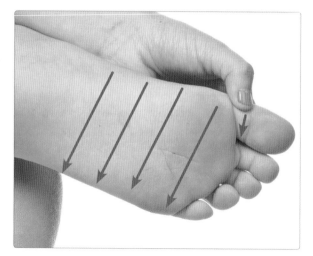

Using the pad of the thumb, gently work the base of the big toe, all across the pad of the foot, and the arch.

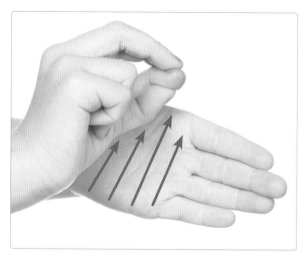

Apply light pressure along the palm side of the thumb, the knuckles where the fingers join the hand, and the whole palm.

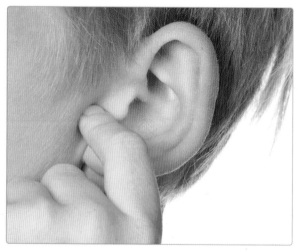

Gently hold the tranquilizer point on the ear.

Ear Infection

Ear infections are all too common in babies and young children. For little ones with ear infections, spend more of your time working on the middle and inner ear reflexes in the hands and feet, and finish by holding the middle and inner ear reflex on the earlobe.

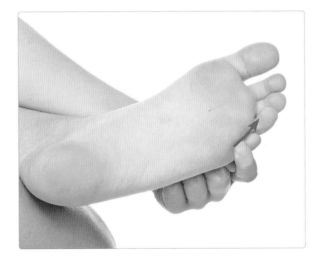

Gently work along the ridge where the base of the two outermost toes join the pad of the foot.

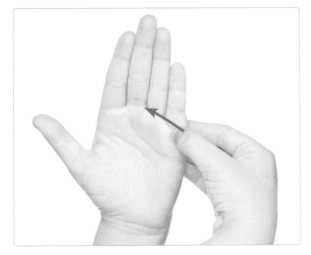

Reflex along the ridge where the base of the two outermost fingers connect to the palm.

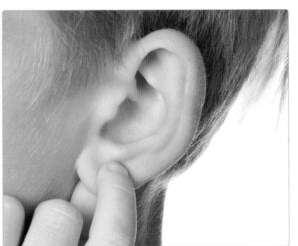

After working on the feet and hands, lightly hold the middle and inner ear reflex on the earlobe.

Reflexology for Seniors

Many countries have legally predetermined ages when a person is considered a senior citizen, ranging from 50 to 65 and upward. Perhaps, instead of a specific age, being a "senior" might be better determined by individual genetics and the quality of life a person has led. Those who have lived wisely, attending to proper sleep, exercise, nutrition, friendships, community service, and so forth, often look and feel much younger, vibrant, and vital than their actual age. And the reverse is also true; those who live hard, abuse their bodies, sleep little, don't exercise, and eat unwisely often look much older than their age.

Either way, some factors are a given. By age 30, many of your body's chemical functions begin to slow down. Your brain, for example, produces fewer feel-good and mental-alertness chemicals, and the same is true for your thyroid, adrenal glands, ovaries or testes, and most of your body's other chemical producers. These changes continue, and their cumulative effect is felt more into your 50, 60, 70s, and beyond. Because of these changes, eventually, you might not be able to sleep as well, take longer to get to sleep, and wake up in the middle of the night and not be able to get back to sleep again. A common problem is the need to urinate more frequently, which is often accompanied by the feeling that your bladder is not empty, or actual loss of bladder control. Dysphagia, or trouble swallowing, can lead to difficulty swallowing foods, liquids, and medicines, or can lead to these things getting stuck in your throat. Other issues like lack of moistness in the eyes, lower libido, difficulty with bowel movements, low energy, cold hands and feet, reduced range of motion and mobility, and more can occur in later years, too.

The aging process, in a sense, is part of the process of life. The question is, do you take the best care of yourself? Is there something else you we can do to prevent or at least minimize some of the effects of aging? To answer that question, let me tell you a story.

Lotti, a lovely petite elderly lady, came to my office wanting regular reflexology sessions. She was very familiar with reflexology, having read and practiced reflexology on herself for decades. However, now she had reached an age when she was becoming frail and didn't have the strength in her hands to do as much self-help reflexology as she used to. Although frail, she still had a wonderful disposition, and she wanted to keep her health, quality of life, sense of well-being, and independence for as long as possible. That's why she came for reflexology sessions, which she did for years, until she could no longer take the bus to my office.

During the last years of her life, Lotti enjoyed a better, more consistent quality of life, thanks to reflexology. She is a wonderful example of a senior maintaining the highest quality of life possible, using regular reflexology as part of the process.

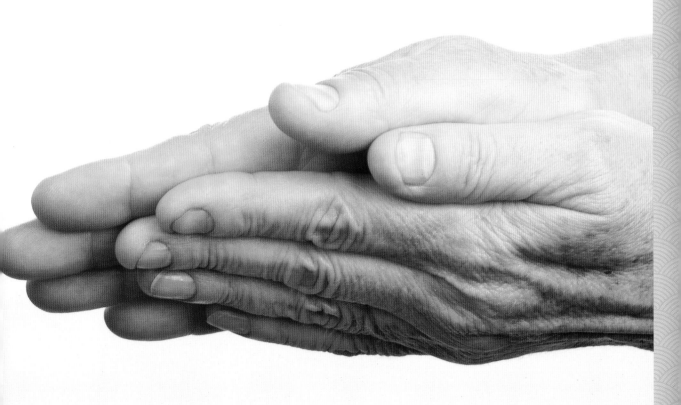

Poor Circulation in the Hands and Feet

Poor blood circulation in the extremities can cause many problems for seniors. To combat this, you can work on specific reflexes for the hands and feet. Additionally, you can work on the reflex points for the arms and legs to better help circulation to and from your hands and feet.

If you have poor circulation in your hands and arms:

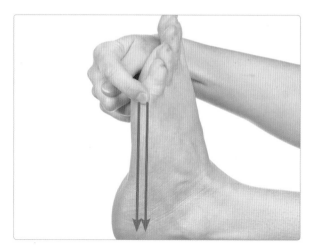

Index finger roll along the outer edge of your foot, from the base of your little toe to below your ankle bone.

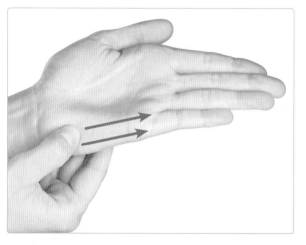

Work along the outer edge of your hand, from near your wrist to below your little finger.

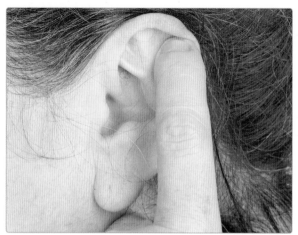

On your ear, gently reflex the upper two thirds of the outer valley and then hold the hand reflex.

If you have poor circulation in your feet and legs:

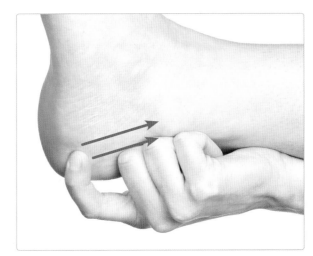

On your feet, index finger roll along the outer edge of your foot below and in front of your ankle bone.

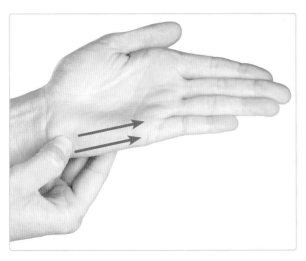

Work all along the outer edge of your hand near your wrist.

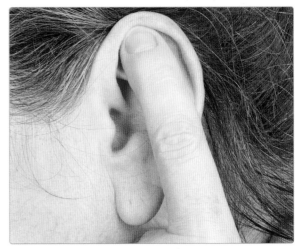

Reflex the entire wide ridge of your ear and then hold your foot reflex.

Insomnia

Many people suffer from insomnia, especially seniors. Reflexing the arch of the foot and the soft palm of the hand can be soothing and help your body relax so you can get to sleep.

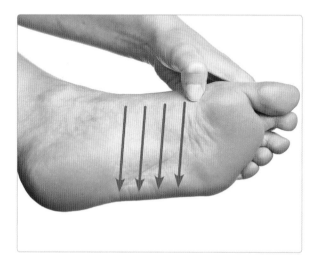

Apply gentle, even pressure all along the arch of your foot.

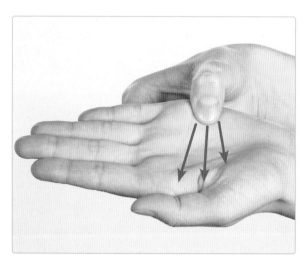

Reflex across the soft part of the palm of your hand.

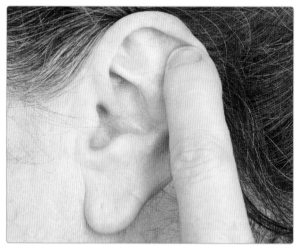

Hold the sleep disorders point on your ear.

Difficulty Swallowing (Dysphagia)

Dysphagia can occur in anyone, but it's more common in seniors. (It's sometimes a problem for infants, too.) For relief, focus on your throat reflex.

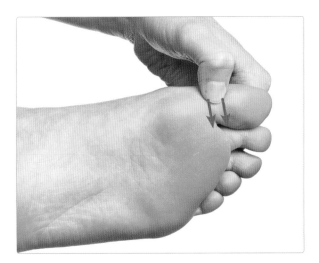

On your feet, thumb roll across the bottom half of your big toe.

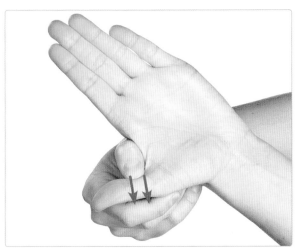

Working on the palm side of your thumb, thumb roll across the base of your thumb, closest to your palm (not the tip).

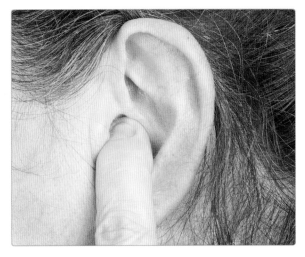

Using the tip of your index finger, hold the throat reflex in your ear.

Frequent Urination

The need to use the restroom more often than usual can be disruptive, whether it occurs during the day or the night. Working the urinary bladder reflex on your foot several times a day, for about 10 minutes each time, can be especially helpful.

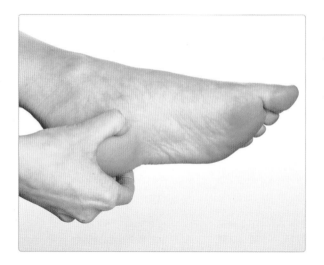

Use a high thumb roll on the urinary bladder reflex on your foot.

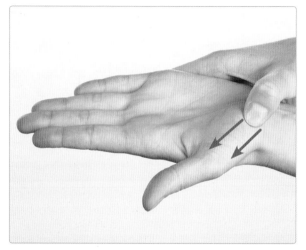

Reflex the inner edge of your hand, near your wrist.

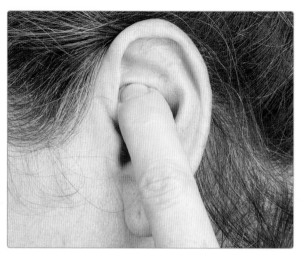

On your ear, apply gentle pressure to the upper part of the upper valley.

Incontinence

The loss of bladder control can be frustrating and embarrassing, no matter what your age. But you can find relief by reflexing your urinary bladder reflex. Repeat this session several times a day, for about 10 minutes each time, for best results.

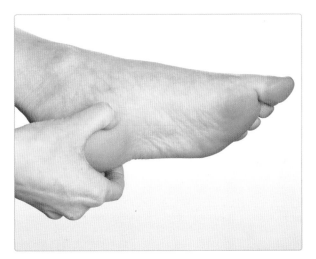

On your foot, thumb roll on your urinary bladder reflex.

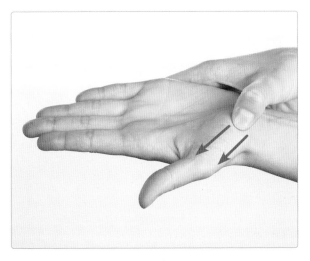

Reflex near your wrist, along the inner edge of your hand.

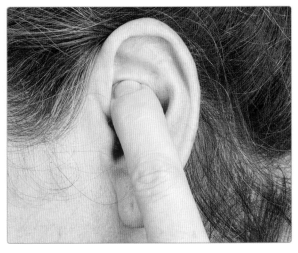

Gently hold the upper part of your ear's upper valley.

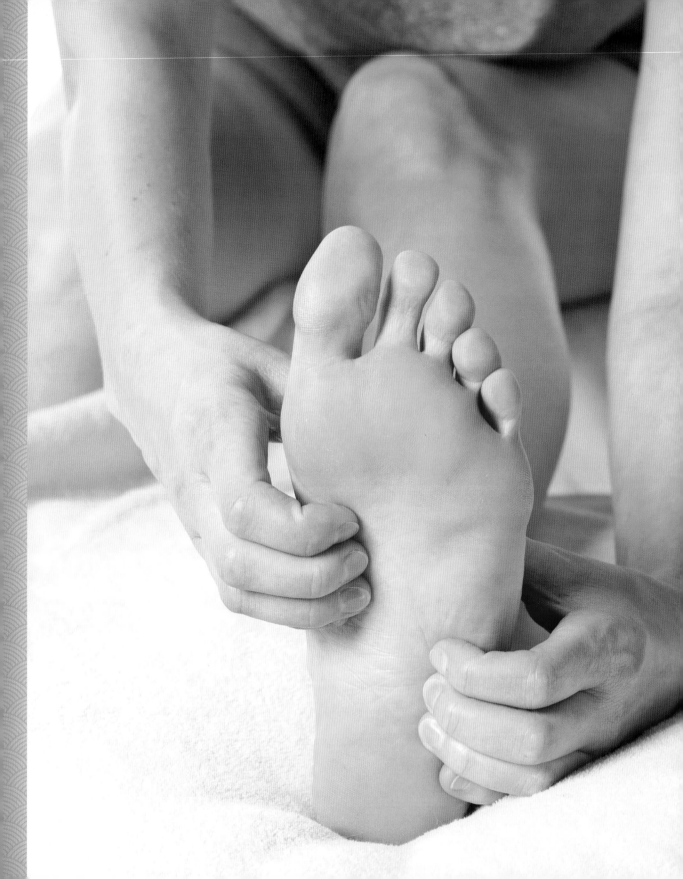

Part 8

Reflexology for Relief

Your body is an absolutely amazing, staggeringly complex, self-healing mechanism. When you treat it well, it treats you well in return. If you are less attentive about your health, your body can be remarkably forgiving ... but only for a while. Eventually, it will send you messages it needs special attention, through aches, ailments, and myriad other symptoms. Using all three—foot, hand, and ear reflexology—on yourself, over a period of sessions, can not only help ease your discomforts, but also reduce or eliminate other symptoms. More importantly, reflexology can help your body do what it was born to do—heal itself.

Part 8 contains a wide range of alphabetical health issues that can plague almost anyone, of any age, and the foot, hand, and ear reflexology work that can help you find relief.

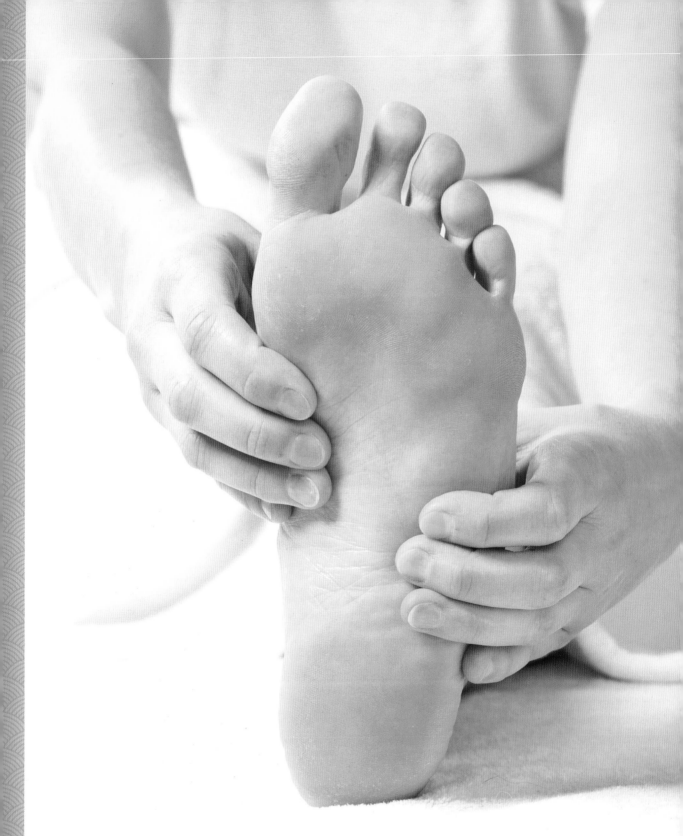

Adrenal Fatigue

Many people suffer from fatigued adrenal glands. Possible symptoms include tiredness, difficulty concentrating, and craving sweet or salty foods, among others. For relief, work on the adrenal reflexes on your feet and hands, and hold the adrenal reflex on your ear.

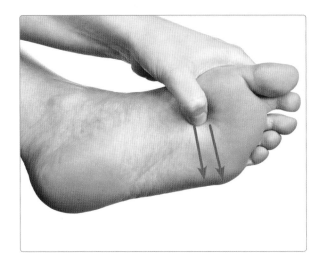

Reflex your upper arch.

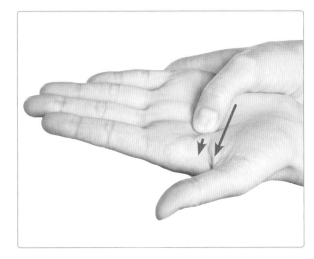

Work the upper part of your palm.

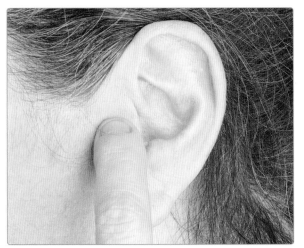

On your ear, hold your facial ridge.

Allergies

Your liver helps break down chemical compounds in your body, especially those related to allergies. So when your allergies are bothering you, work your liver reflexes. The allergy point on your ears can help reduce allergic symptoms such as those from pollen, topical substances, and pet dander.

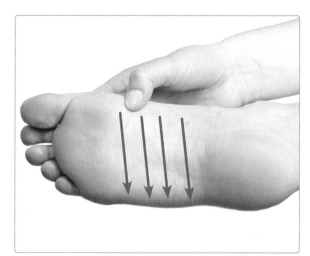

Reflex along the arch of your right foot, and move to your left foot.

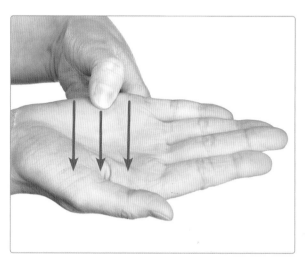

Work on the soft palm of your right hand, and switch to your left hand for a while.

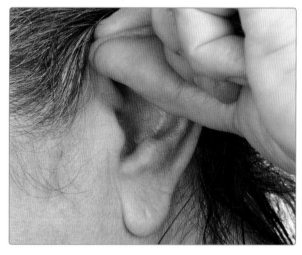

Hold the allergy point at the top of your ear's outer ridge.

Ankle Pain

Working on the ankle reflexes on your feet, hands, and ears can dramatically reduce or eliminate ankle pain. If your pain persists, however, make an appointment with your physician to have it checked.

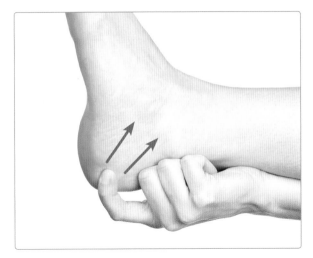

Gently work along the outer edge of your ankle, below your ankle bone.

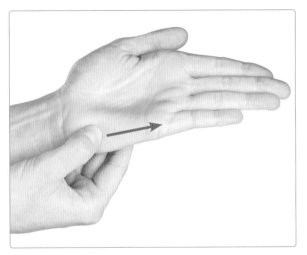

On your hand, reflex the outer edge, near your wrist.

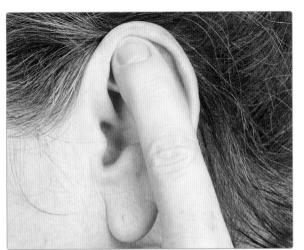

Apply gentle pressure near the top of your ear's wide ridge.

Anxiety

Reflexology can be quite effective at relieving feelings of anxiety. Working the entire bottom of your feet and the palm of your hands and then holding the anxiety point on your ear for 5 minutes at a time, or longer, should help the feelings subside.

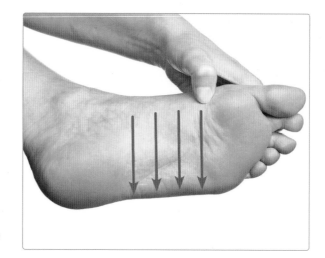

Reflex all along the bottom of your big toe and the arch of your foot.

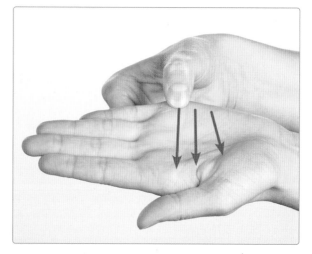

On your hand, work your palm and the palm side of your thumb.

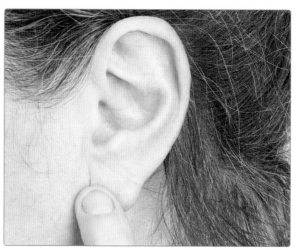

Hold the anxiety point on your earlobe.

Appendicitis

Your appendix, located in your lower-right abdomen, can become inflamed and painful. If you're in severe pain and suspect you have appendicitis, seek medical help immediately. Note that although most reflexology can be done on either or both sides of your body, because your appendix is in your lower-right part of your abdomen, stick to your right foot, hand, and ear when reflexing for appendicitis.

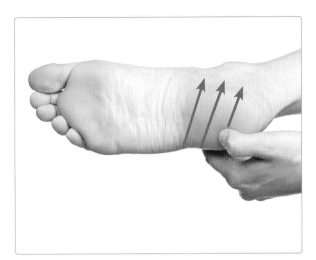

Reflex the arch and heel of your right foot.

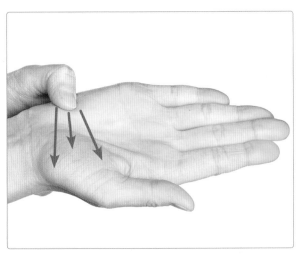

Reflex the soft part of your palm and the heel of your right hand.

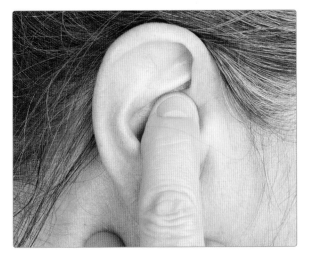

On your right ear, hold your upper valley.

Arthritis

Arthritis can manifest in many bones and joints throughout the body. When seeking relief for arthritis pain, you can target the specific areas that hurt, like your neck, shoulder, or elbow, or you can reflex for everything. Remember, though, when working on arthritic parts of the body to reflex lightly.

If you have arthritis in your neck:

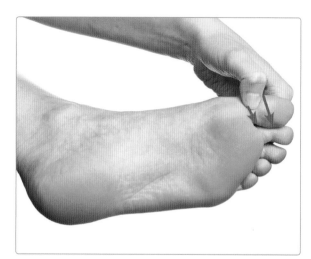

Focusing on your big toe, work along the bottom surface, closest to your foot.

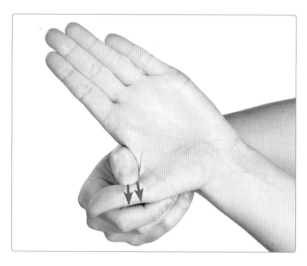

Focusing on your thumb, work along the palm side, closest to your palm.

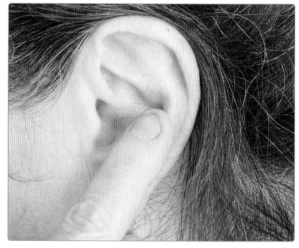

On your ear, hold the lower part of your middle ridge.

If you have arthritis in your shoulder:

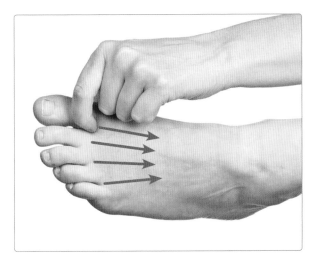

Reflex along the grooves on the top of your foot.

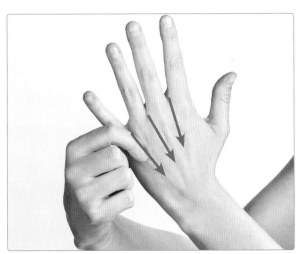

Work along the grooves on the back of your hand.

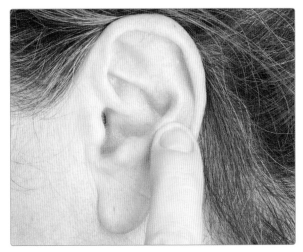

Hold near the bottom of your ear's outer valley.

Arthritis *(continued)*

If you have arthritis in your elbow:

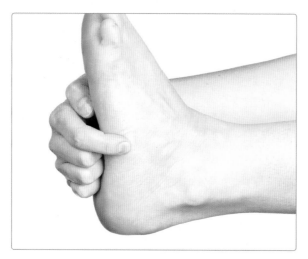

Reflex along the middle-outer edge of your foot.

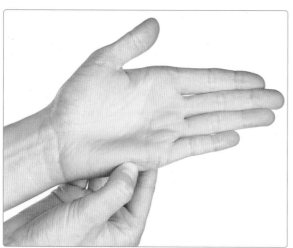

On your hand, work along the middle-outer edge.

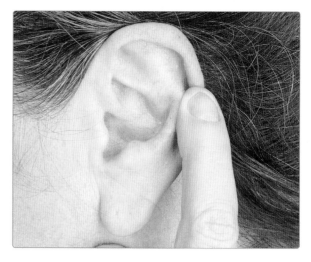

On your ear, hold midway up your outer valley.

If you have arthritis in your wrist:

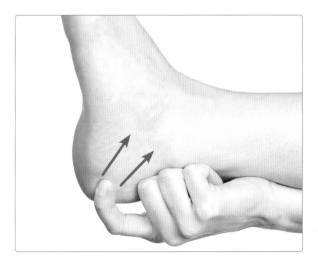

Work the outer edge of your foot, below your ankle bone.

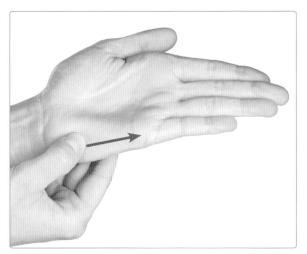

Reflex the outer edge of your hand, near your wrist.

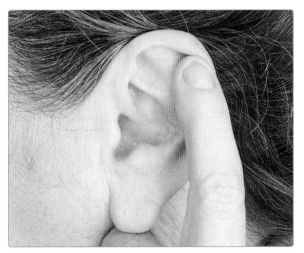

Gently work near the top of your ear's outer valley.

Arthritis *(continued)*

If you have arthritis in your back:

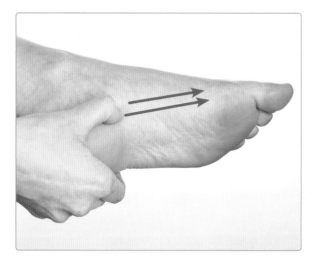

Reflex all along the inner edge of your foot.

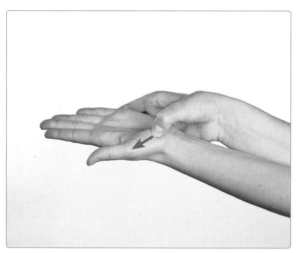

On your hand, also work along the inner edge.

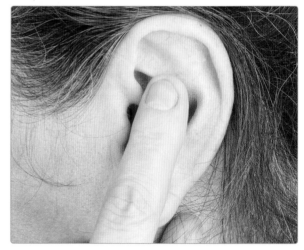

Gently reflex along the middle and narrow ridge of your ear.

If you have arthritis in your hip:

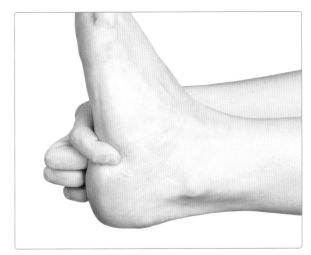

Reflex the outer edge of your foot, below and slightly in front of your ankle bone.

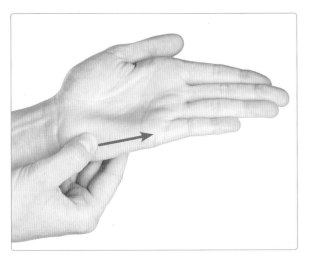

Work all along the outer edge of your hand, near your wrist.

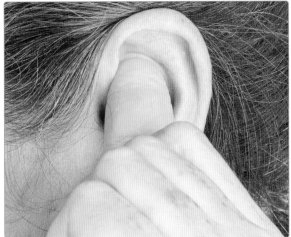

Gently reflex the intersection of your ear's narrow and wide ridges.

Arthritis *(continued)*

If you have arthritis in your knee:

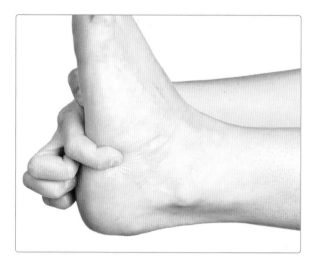

Evenly work along the outer edge of your foot below and in front of your ankle bone.

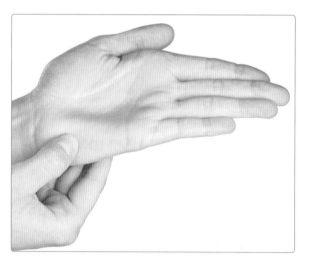

Reflex along the outer edge of your hand, close to your wrist.

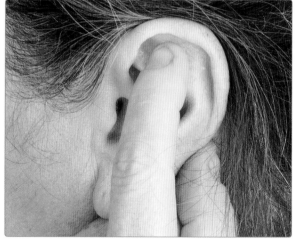

On your ear, gently work midway up your wide ridge.

If you have arthritis in your ankle:

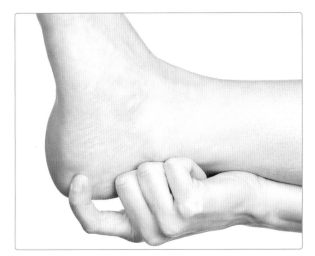

Reflex below your ankle bone, on the outer edge of your foot.

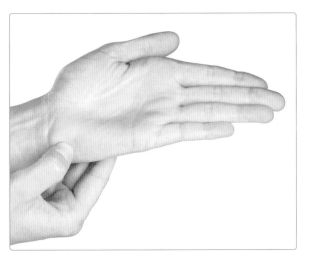

Gently work the outer edge of your hand, near your wrist.

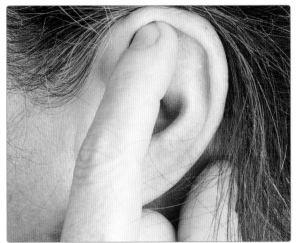

Hold the top of your ear's wide ridge.

Asthma

Anything that affects your breathing can be frightening. If you suffer from asthma, be patient and take your time for best results. An hour of working on your feet, hands, and ears often gradually relieves labored breathing.

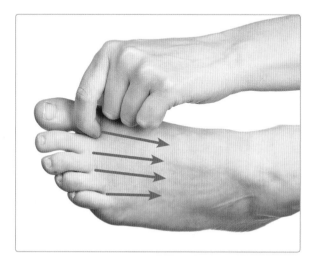

Gently work all along the groves on top of your foot.

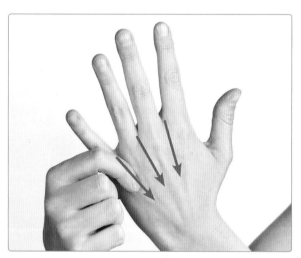

Evenly reflex the grooves on the back of your hand.

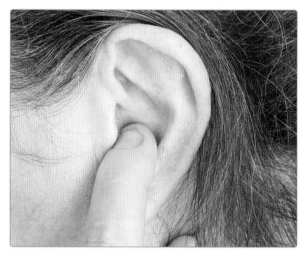

On your ear, hold the center of your lower valley.

Athlete's Foot

The itching and other discomforts that sometimes accompany athlete's foot can be eased with reflexology. Holding the toe and foot reflex at the top of the wide ridge of the ear is especially helpful.

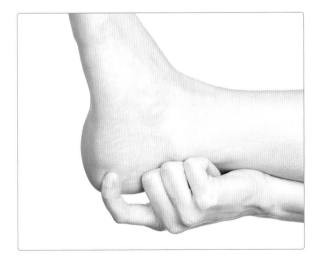

Work along the outer edge of your foot, below your ankle bone.

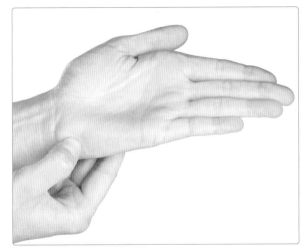

Reflex the outer edge of your hand, near your wrist.

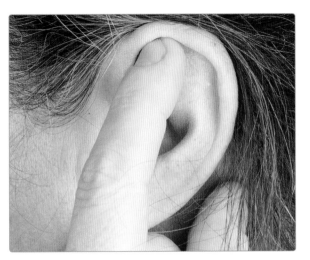

Gently work along the top of your ear's wide ridge.

Back Pain

People all over the world live with back pain. Reflexing the feet is especially helpful for relief of mid back (thoracic vertebrae) pain. Thumb roll, slowly and repeatedly, on your feet and hands, reflexing the tissue from every direction. For relief of lower back pain, hold the narrow ridge on your ear for 10, 20, or even 30 minutes. Also work on the lower back reflexes on your feet and hands.

If you have pain in your mid back:

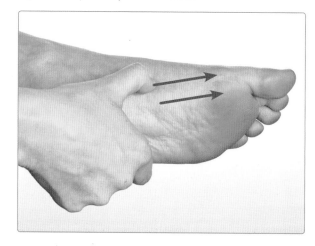

Thumb roll midway along the inner edge of your foot.

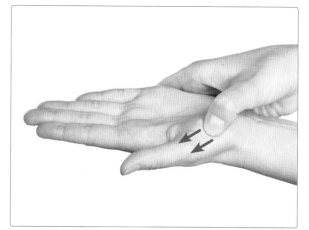

Slowly and repeatedly thumb roll midway along the inner edge of your hand.

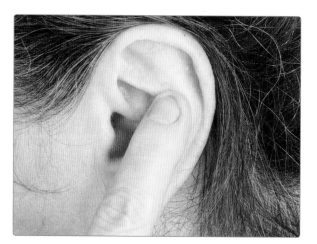

Gently reflex midway up the arch of your middle ridge.

If you have pain in your lower back:

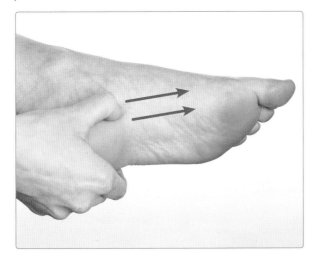

Reflex the inner edge of your foot near where your arch and heel meet.

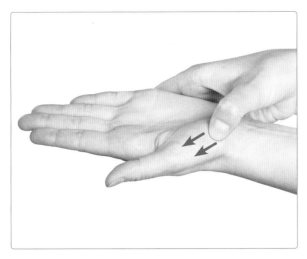

Work on the inner edge of your hand, near your wrist.

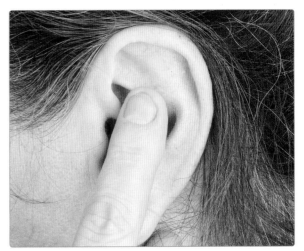

On your ear, gently work on your narrow ridge.

Balance

If you have balance problems, work on your inner ear reflexes for relief. Focus on your hands first before moving to your feet. Then finish by holding the middle and inner ear reflex on your earlobe.

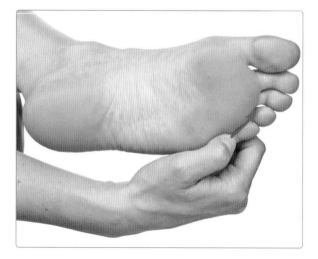

Evenly reflex along the ridge where the base of your two outermost toes connect to your foot.

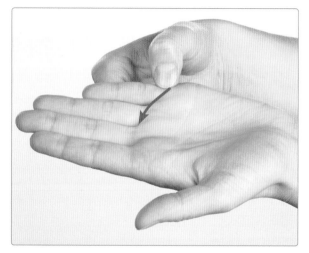

Reflex along the ridge where the base of your two outermost fingers connect to your hand.

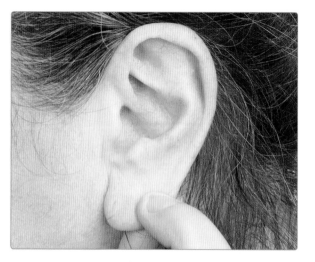

Hold the area slightly back of the middle part of your earlobe.

Bronchitis

If you're suffering from the cough, fever, chest pain, and other symptoms of bronchitis, there is help. Spend most of your time reflexing the grooves on the top of your foot and the back of your hand before moving on to your ear.

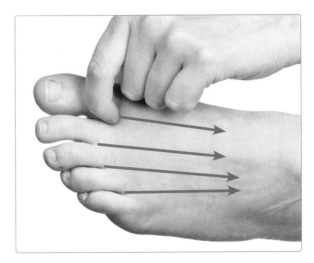

Evenly work the grooves on the top of your foot.

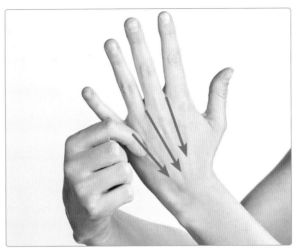

Gently reflex the grooves on the back of your hand.

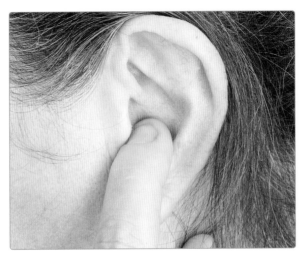

Hold the lung reflex in the center of your ear's lower valley for 5 minutes.

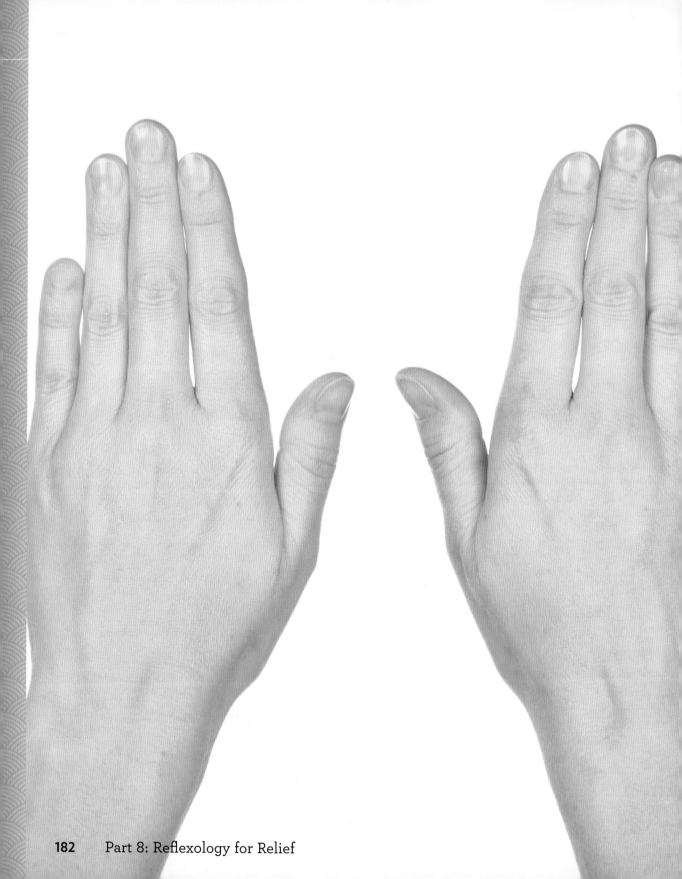

Carpel Tunnel Syndrome

If you have the pain, tingling, and numbness often associated with carpel tunnel syndrome, you want to avoid making things worse, so don't directly touch a sore forearm, wrist, or hand. Instead, reflex the forearm and hand points on your hands, feet, and ears.

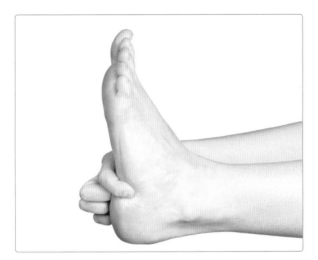

Reflex the outer edge of your foot, below your ankle bone.

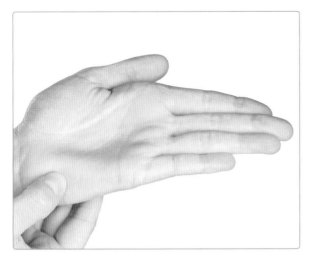

Gently work along the outer edge of your hand, near your wrist.

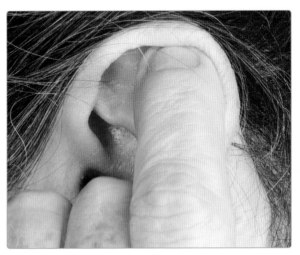

Apply pressure to the upper third of your ear's outer valley.

Cold

Unfortunately, there's no cure for the common cold, but reflexology can help relieve your symptoms. Be careful to not work deeply, however. Doing so can release toxins, which could make you feel even worse. Work lightly, especially on your hands and feet.

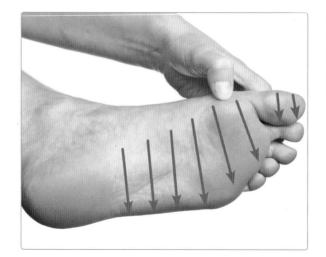

Reflex your big toe, the ball and pad of your foot, and the arch.

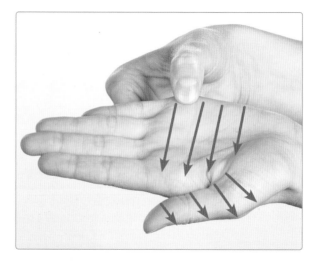

Work your thumb, your big knuckles, and the soft part of your palm.

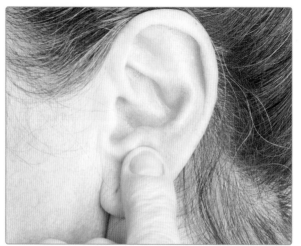

Gently reflex your earlobe as well as your ear's lower and upper valleys.

Constipation

When you're suffering from constipation, you can feel stuck. But relief is available. Powerful reflexing of your arch and heel can help get things moving again. Start with medium pressure on your feet and hands, and gradually apply deeper pressure.

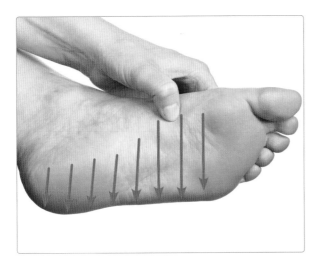

Deeply and evenly work your arch and heel.

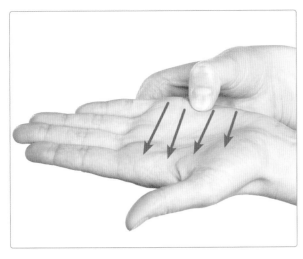

Apply even pressure all over the palm of your hand.

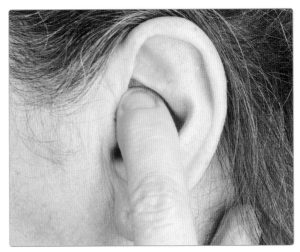

On your ear, hold the upper part of your upper valley.

Crohn's Disease

Crohn's disease, or inflammation in the digestive tract, can be painful and uncomfortable. It can occur anywhere in your lower digestive tract, but it's usually in your lower-right abdomen. Spending some time reflexing your right foot, hand, and ear can provide relief.

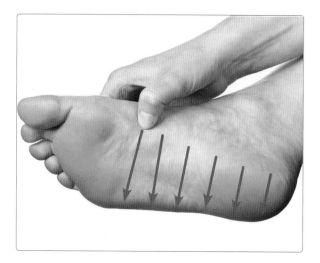

Gently reflex your arch and heel.

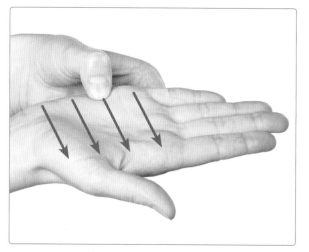

On your hand, work all along your palm.

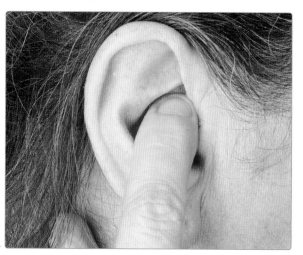

Press and hold the upper part of your ear's upper valley.

Depression

For those who live with depression, it can be a debilitating condition. When the brain doesn't produce enough of the necessary chemicals to adequately buoy you, reflexology can provide some relief. Spend lots of time gently reflexing the outer half of your toes and fingers, and hold the antidepression point on your ear for 5 minutes at a time.

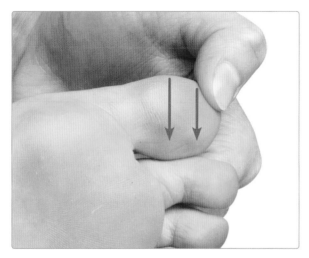

Gently reflex the outer half of the bottom side of your big toe.

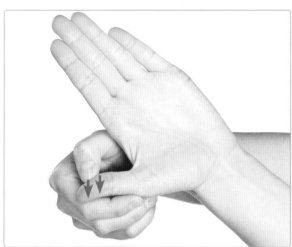

Evenly work along the outer half of the palm side of your thumb.

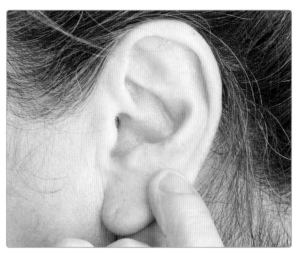

Gently hold the antidepression point on your earlobe, just below the base of your middle ridge.

Diabetes

When your body can't properly control the amount of glucose, or sugar, it contains due to a shortfall of insulin, diabetes can result. Because insulin is produced in the pancreas, that's where you should focus your reflexology work. Although the head of the pancreas is on your right side, most of the organ is on your left, behind your stomach, so spend most of your time reflexing your left foot, hand, and ear.

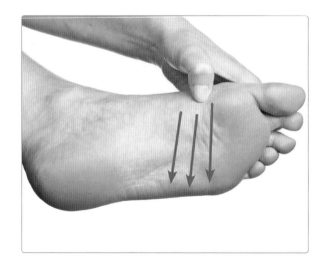

Gently work the arch of your left foot and switch to your right arch for awhile.

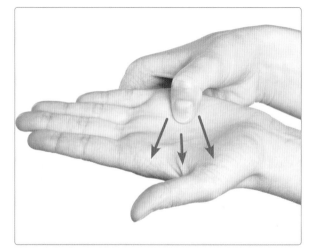

On your hands, work the palm of your left hand and move to your right hand for a bit.

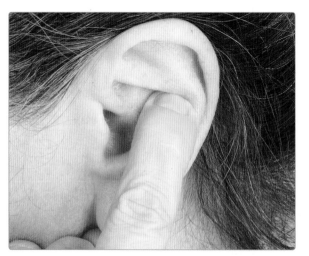

On your ear, hold the beginning of the upper valley.

Diarrhea

When suffering the discomfort of diarrhea, spend some time reflexing your feet and hands and then move to the colon reflex in your ear. Also, remember to drink plenty of fluids to avoid the risk of dehydration.

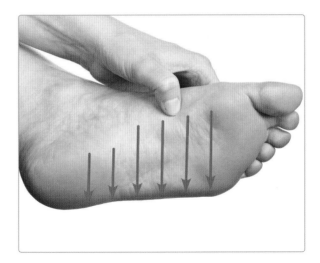

Take time to work your arch and your heel.

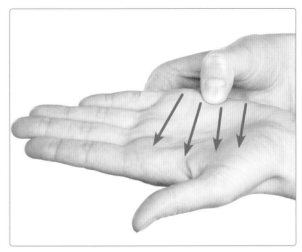

Reflex the soft palm and heel of your hand.

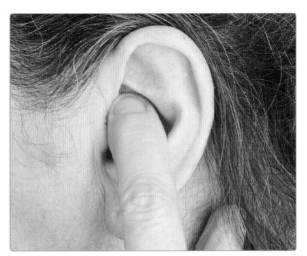

Hold the colon reflex in your ear's upper valley.

Digestive Problems

Most digestive upsets occur in your upper and lower abdomen, but you also might experience some discomfort in your chest if you have acid reflux. Depending on where your symptoms are, you can target specific points to reflex, or you can reflex for everything.

If you have digestive upset in your chest:

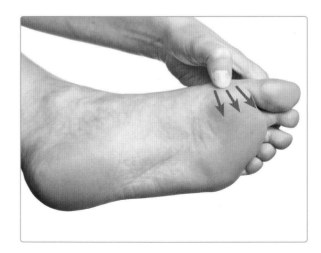

Reflex the ball-shape knuckle below your big toe.

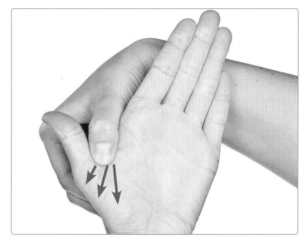

Work the big knuckle at the base of your thumb.

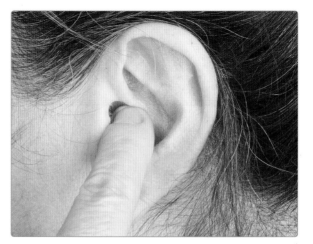

On your ear, hold the upper part of your lower valley.

If you have digestive upset in your upper abdomen:

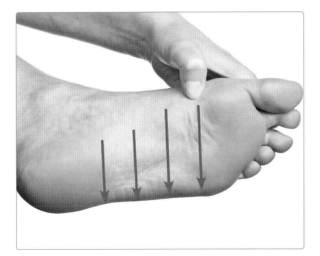

Evenly work all along the arch of your foot.

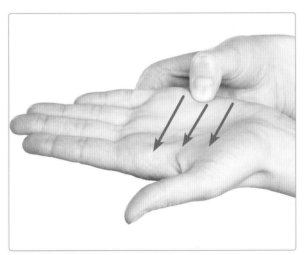

Work all over the soft parts of your palm.

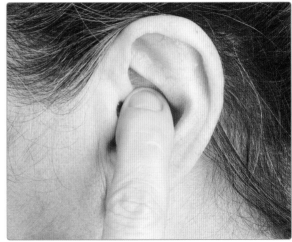

On your ear, work your upper valley.

Digestive Problems *(continued)*

If you have digestive upset in your lower abdomen:

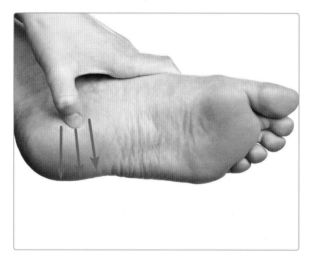

Work all over
your heel.

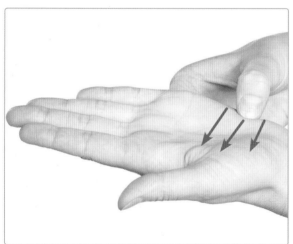

Spend some time reflexing the heel of your palm.

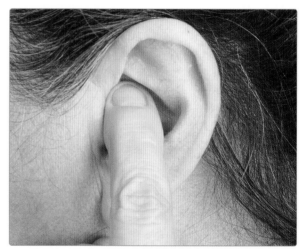

On your ear, gently work your upper valley.

Diverticulitis

Diverticulitis can cause abdominal pain, nausea, and a host of other issues. The condition can occur anywhere in your digestive system, but it most often presents in the sigmoid colon, in the lower-left abdomen. For relief, spend more time on your left foot, hand, and ear.

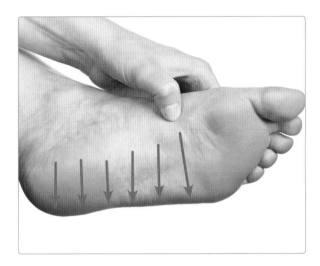

Work on the lower arch and heel of your left foot.

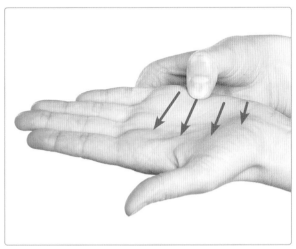

Reflex the soft palm and heel of your left hand.

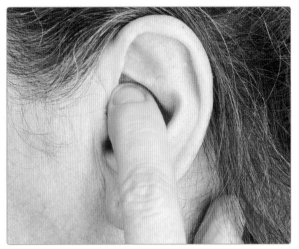

Hold the upper part of your upper valley.

Dizziness

When you suffer from dizziness, usually your inner ear is to blame. Spend more of your time working on the middle and inner ear reflexes on your hands, work the same areas on your feet, and finish by holding the middle and inner ear reflex on your earlobe.

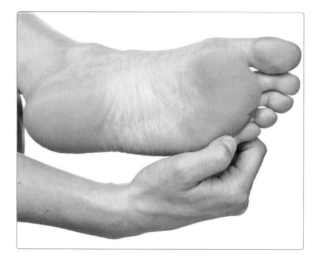

Reflex the ridge where the base of your two outermost toes connect to your foot.

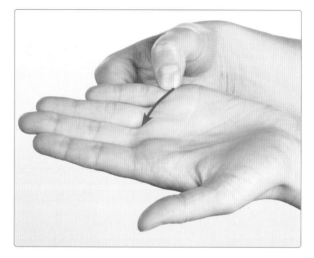

Work along the ridge where the base of your ring and little finger connect to your hand.

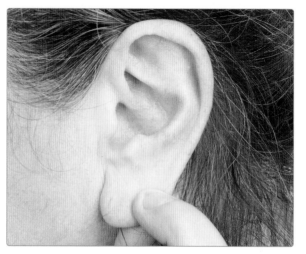

On your ear, hold the point slightly back of the middle part of your earlobe.

Earache

Earaches most frequently occur in children, but adults can experience ear pain or pressure, too. For relief, spend more of your time working on the middle and inner ear reflexes in your hands, move to your feet, and finish by holding the middle and inner ear reflex on your earlobe.

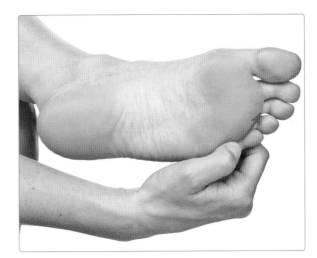

Reflex the ridge where the base of your two outermost toes connect to the pad of your foot.

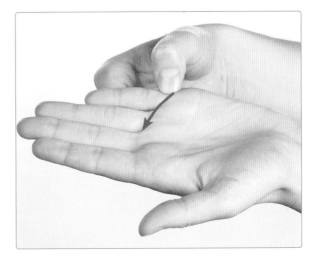

Work on the ridge where the base of your two outermost fingers connect to the palm of your hand.

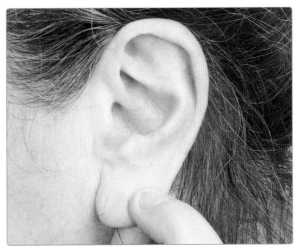

Hold slightly back from the middle part of your earlobe.

Eczema

Itchy, uncomfortable eczema (atopic dermatitis) can occur on your skin anywhere on your body. This irritating rash, or inflammation, can flare up and go away often. For relief of the discomfort it causes, you can target specific areas to reflex, or you can reflex for everything. However, avoid working directly on skin that's inflamed.

If you have eczema on your head:

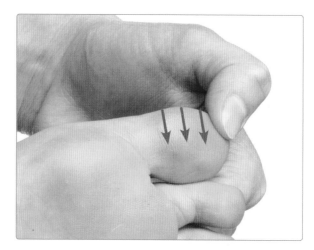

Reflex the outside of the bottom of your big toe.

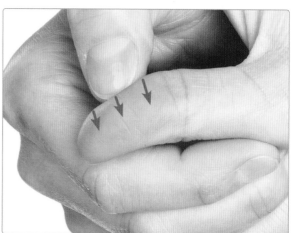

Work on the outside half of your thumb, on the palm side.

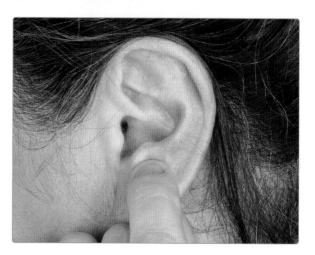

Gently work your upper earlobe.

If you have eczema on your neck:

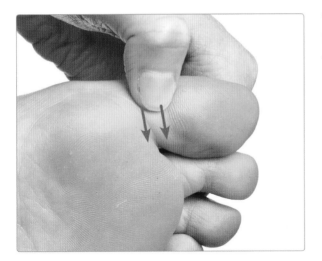

Work on the
lower half of
your big toe.

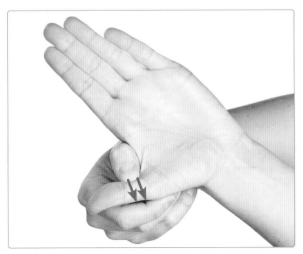

On the palm side of your thumb, reflex the half
closest to your hand.

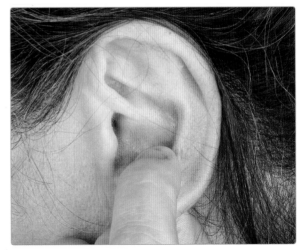

On your ear, reflex the lower part of your middle
ridge.

Eczema *(continued)*

If you have eczema on your chest:

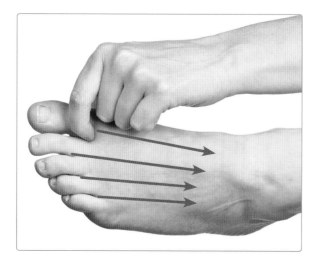

Reflex the grooves on the top of your foot.

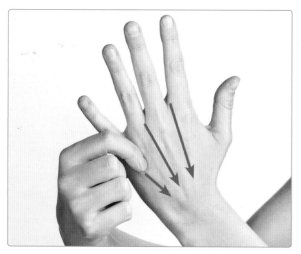

Gently work on the grooves on the back of your hand.

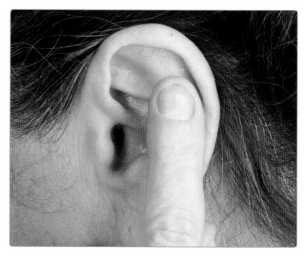

On your ear, reflex halfway up your middle ridge.

If you have eczema on your back:

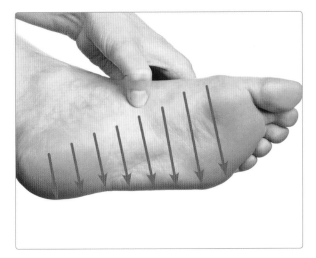

Reflex the inner edge of your foot as well as your arch and your heel.

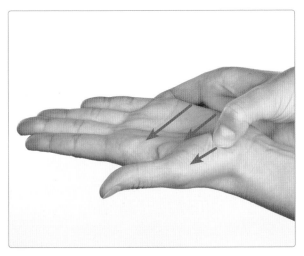

On your hand, work on the inner edge, the palm, and the heel.

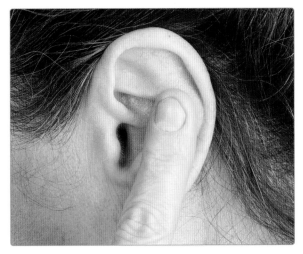

Work on the upper two thirds of the middle ridge of your ear.

Eczema *(continued)*

If you have eczema on your arms:

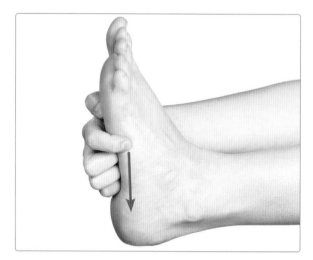

Reflex the outer edge of your foot.

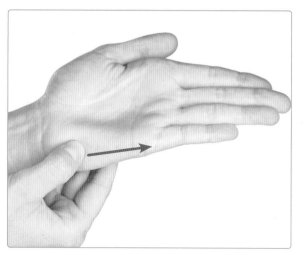

Work along the outer edge of your hand.

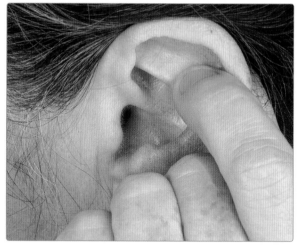

Gently reflex the upper two thirds of your outer valley.

If you have eczema on your legs:

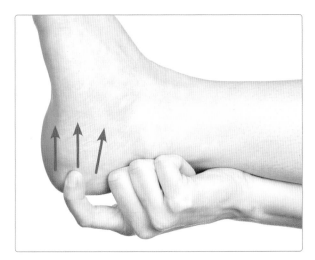

Work along the outer edge of your foot, below and in front of your ankle bone.

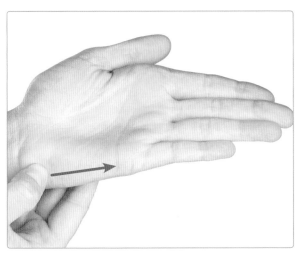

Reflex the outer edge of your hand, near your wrist.

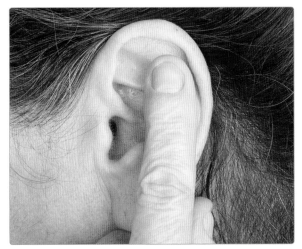

On your ear, gently work on your wide ridge.

Elbow Pain

Elbow pain can be caused by many things, but for relief of some of the most common causes of pain or discomfort in this joint, work on the elbow reflex in the outer edge of your hand for a while, move to the elbow reflex on your foot, and finish by working on the elbow reflex in your ear.

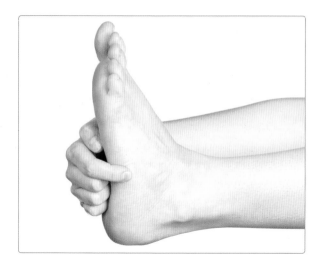

Reflex at about the midway point on the outer edge of your foot.

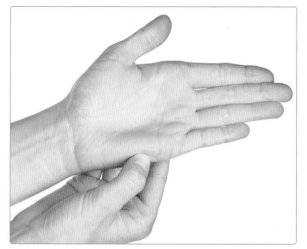

On your hand, reflex at about the midway point on the outer edge.

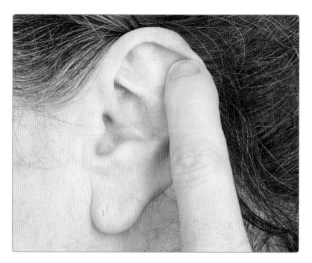

Gently hold the spot about halfway up your ear's outer valley.

Emphysema

Emphysema, one of the chronic obstructive pulmonary diseases (COPDs), usually is caused by the breakdown of the walls of the tiny little air sacs in the lungs, making it difficult for you to get enough oxygen. Working grooves on the tops of your feet and the backs of your hands can help your lungs relax and make breathing easier.

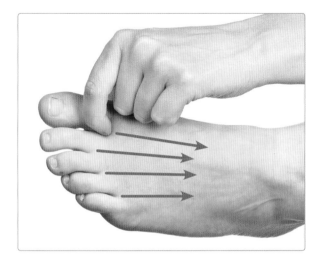

Reflex the grooves on the top of your foot.

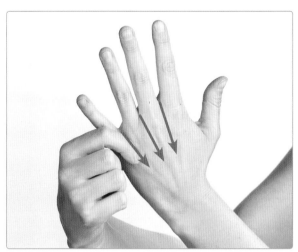

Reflex the grooves on the back of your hand.

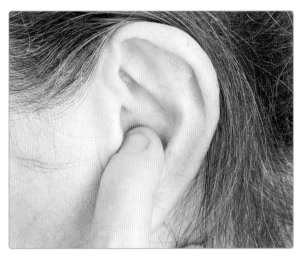

On your ear, hold the center part of your lower valley.

Eyestrain

Eyestrain occurs when your eyes are fatigued from extensive use, especially when you're looking at a fixed point for a period of time. To ease eyestrain discomfort, work the part of the ridge at the base of your fingers and toes.

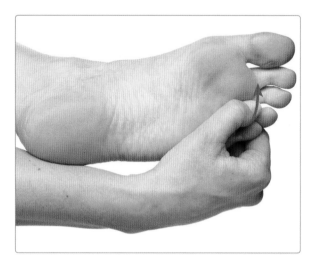

Reflex the ridge where the base of your second and third toes connect to the pad of your foot.

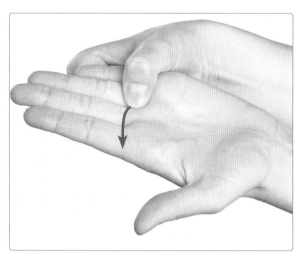

Work on the ridge where the base of your middle and index fingers connect to your palm.

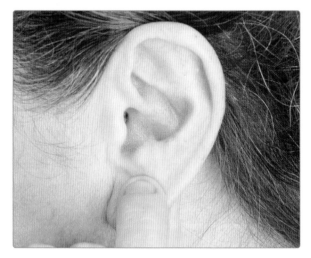

Hold the middle of your earlobe.

Fatigue

For relief of temporary fatigue, or tiredness, reflex for everything from your head, neck, and shoulders, down to your lower abdomen. Repeated several times a week, this reflexology work can help give your system the rest it needs.

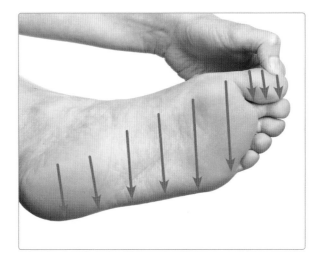

Reflex the bottom side of your big toe and the bottom of your foot.

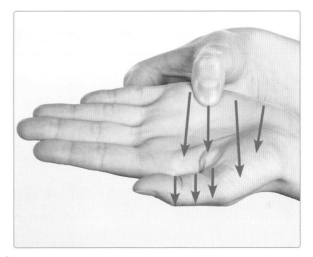

Work the palm side of your thumb and the palm of your hand.

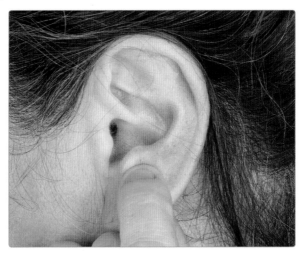

On your ear, gently work on the upper part of your earlobe and the lower part of your inner ridge.

Flu

When you're suffering from the fever, congestion, cough, and overall achy feeling the flu can cause, you need relief. Reflex lightly, especially on your hands and feet. Be careful to not work deeply because doing so can release toxins—which could make you feel even worse!

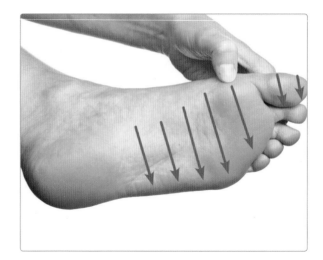

Reflex your big toe, the ball and pad of your foot, and your arch.

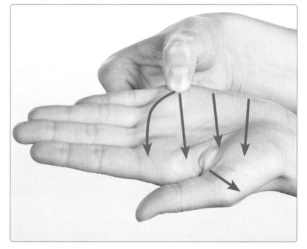

Reflex your thumb, your large knuckles at the base of your fingers, and the soft part of your palm.

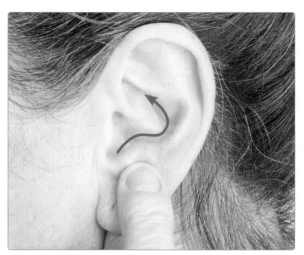

On your ear, reflex your earlobe as well as your lower and upper valleys.

Gallstone

Your gallbladder stores bile from your liver before it's moved along into your intestine to aid in digestion. Within your gallbladder, painful gallstones can form. For relief, spend extra time reflexing the arch of your foot and the soft part of your palm. Note that although most reflexology work is applicable to either or both sides of your body, because your gallbladder sits in the upper-right part of your abdomen, stick to your right foot, hand, and ear when reflexing for gallstones.

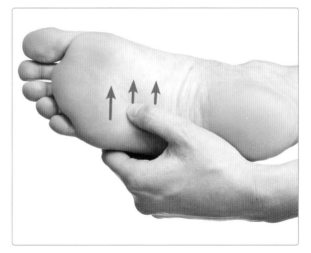

Reflex near the center of the arch of your right foot.

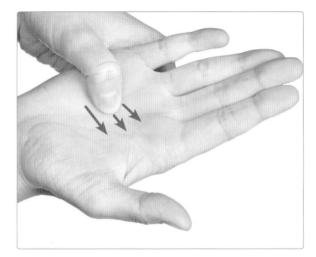

Reflex near the center of the soft part of your right palm.

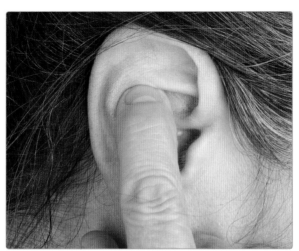

On your right ear, firmly hold the upper valley near the middle ridge.

Glaucoma

Glaucoma is an eye disease caused by a high pressure inside your eye that can damage your optic nerve and may result in loss of vision. For relief of discomfort associated with glaucoma, work at the base of your fingers and toes.

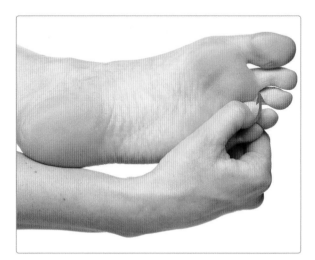

Reflex the ridge where your second and third toes connect to the pad of your foot.

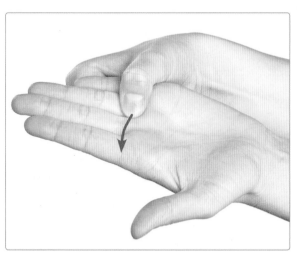

Reflex the ridge where the base of your middle and index fingers connect to your palm.

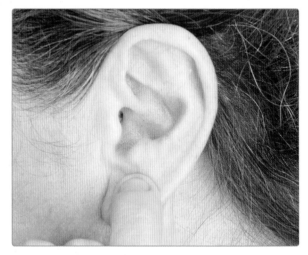

On your ear, hold the middle of your earlobe.

Hay Fever

Living with the itchy eyes, runny nose, sneezing, and sinus pressure hay fever brings can make you miserable. For relief, spend some time holding the allergy point on the top overhang of your ear's outer ridge before moving on to the grooves on the top of your feet and the back of your hands.

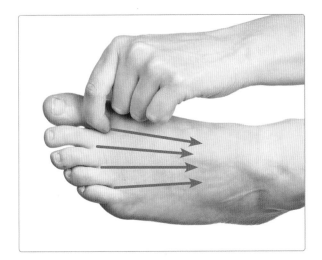

Reflex the grooves on top of your foot.

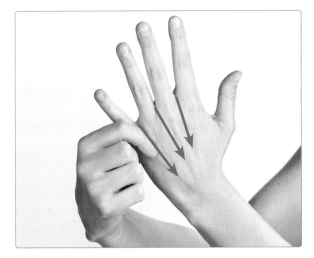

Work the grooves on the back of your hand.

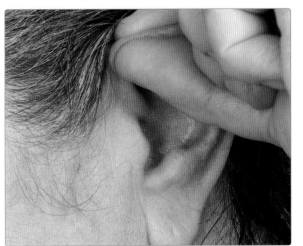

Hold the allergy point at the top of your ear's outer ridge.

Headache

In addition to being painful, headaches can be distracting, especially when one is so bad, you can't think of anything else. For quickest relief, hold the brain reflex on the upper part of your earlobe, just below your lobe ridge, until your headache starts getting better. Then proceed to your big toe, followed by your thumb.

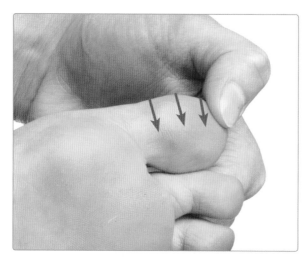

Reflex the outer half of the bottom side of your big toe.

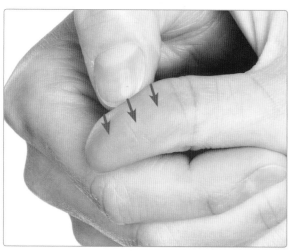

Work on the outer half of the palm-side surface of your thumb.

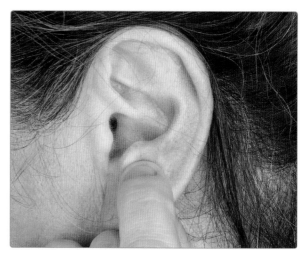

On your ear, reflex the upper center of your earlobe.

Heartburn

When you have burning pain in your chest, it's difficult to concentrate on anything else. For relief of heartburn pain, work on the arch of your left foot and the soft palm of your left hand. Then, hold the stomach reflex on your left ear.

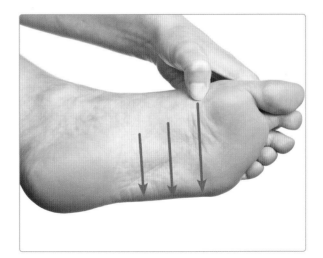

Reflex the arch of your left foot.

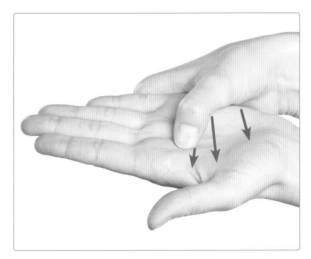

On your left hand, reflex the soft part of your palm.

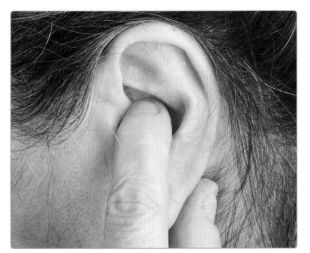

On your left ear, hold the middle ridge near the root of the outer ridge.

Heel Spur

Heel spurs are hard, sometimes painful growths on the heel of your foot. For relief of the pain associated with heel spurs, hold the heel reflex on the wide ridge in your ear. To reduce the recurrence of heel spurs, gently reflex the heel of your foot from every direction before moving on to reflex your hand.

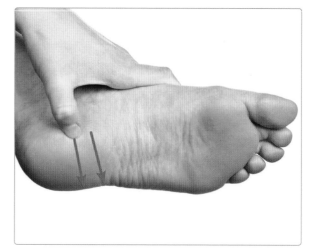

On your foot, gently reflex above and below the imaginary line that runs between your arch and your heel.

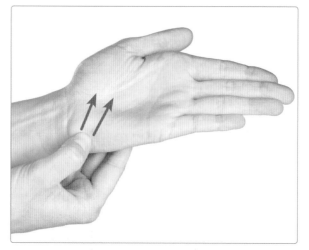

Work above and below the imaginary line that runs between the soft part of your palm and the heel of your hand.

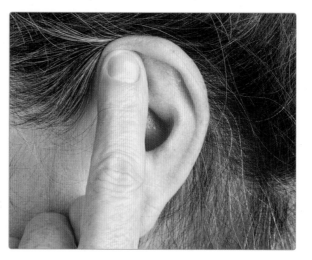

On your ear, reflex the top of the wide ridge, near the triangular valley.

Hemorrhoid

Hemorrhoids can occur in nearly anyone, but they're especially common in older adults and pregnant women. For relief of the discomfort hemorrhoids can cause, reflex the area behind your heel bone, below your Achilles tendon. Use the bony tips of your fingers or the tip of your thumb for best results.

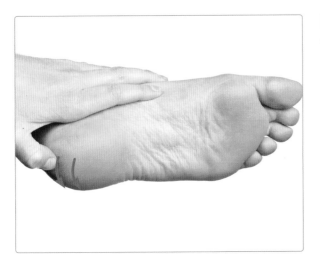

Reflex the back of your heel.

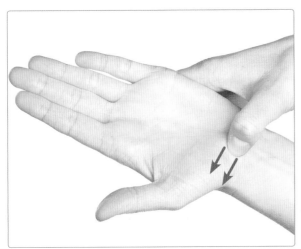

Reflex below the heel part of your palm.

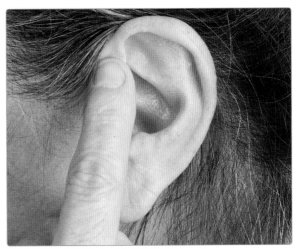

On your ear, hold the outer ridge, near the narrow ridge.

Hernia

Two common types of hernia are hiatal and inguinal. A hiatal hernia occurs in the upper-left abdomen, where the esophagus connects with the top of the stomach. Inguinal hernias most commonly happen in men and manifest as a weakness in the lower abdominal wall that can lead to the intestines pushing through. This, then, can lead to a bulge and often causes substantial pain. Although you want to reflex for both sides of the body, spend more time working on the side of the body where the hernia is.

If you have a hiatal hernia:

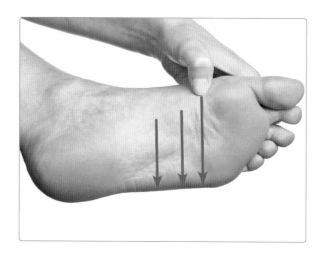

Reflex the arch of your left foot.

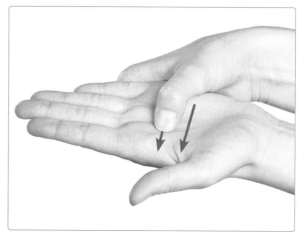

Work on the soft part of the palm of your left hand.

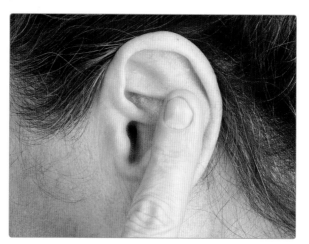

On your left ear, hold the middle ridge.

If you have an inguinal hernia:

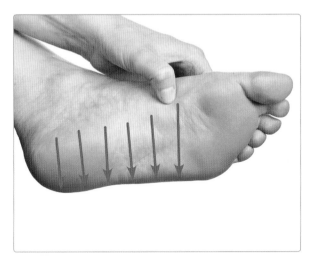

Reflex all along your arch and your heel.

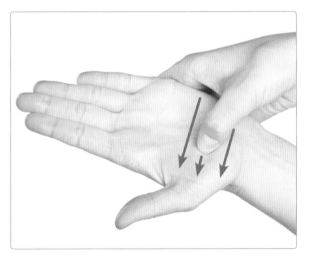

Work on the soft part of the palm of your hand as well as the heel of your hand.

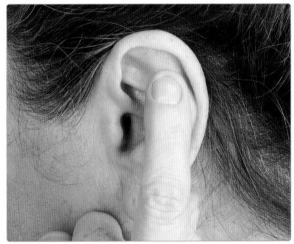

Reflex the upper part of the middle ridge in your ear.

Hiccups

Hiccups occur when your diaphragm, the large muscle that runs below your lungs and above your stomach, spasms. Working deep into the soft part of the palm of your left hand, near your big knuckles, can bring dramatic relief of hiccups. Be sure to also work on your left foot, and hold the stomach reflex on your left ear.

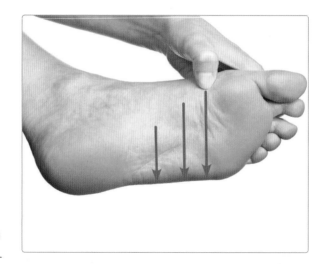

Reflex the arch of your left foot.

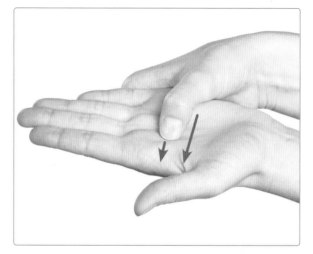

Reflex the soft part of the palm of your left hand.

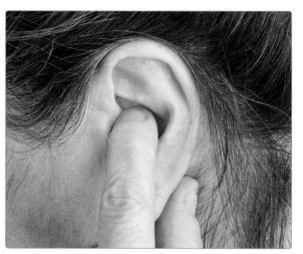

On your left ear, hold the middle ridge, near the root of the outer ridge.

High Blood Pressure

If you have hypertension, or high blood pressure, hold the hypertension point in the highest part of your ear's triangular valley. Then, be sure to spend some time working on the heart reflexes on your feet and hands as well.

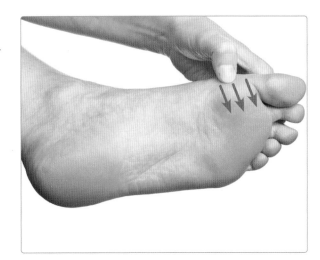

On your foot, reflex the ball at base of your big toe.

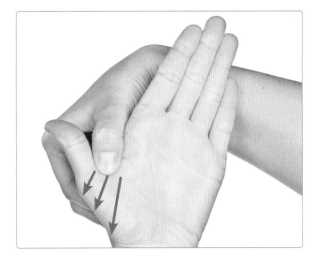

Reflex the big knuckle at the base of your thumb.

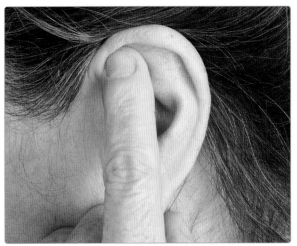

Hold the hypertension point in the upper part of your ear's triangular valley.

Hip Pain

Hip pain can occur for a variety of reasons in a variety of people, although it seems to be more common in older adults and often athletes. For relief, spend some time index finger rolling on the area in front of and below your outer ankle, move to your hands, and then hold the leg reflex in your ear.

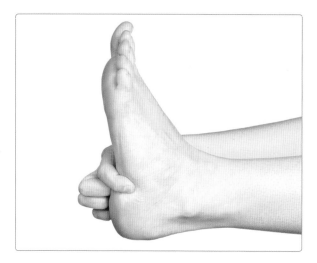

Reflex the outer edge of your ankle, below and slightly in front of your ankle bone.

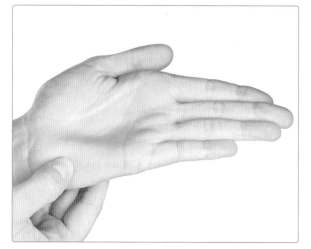

Work along the outer edge of your hand, near your wrist.

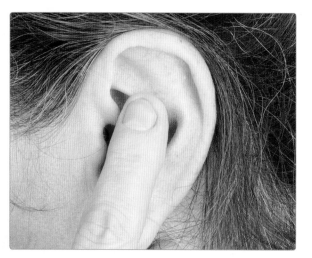

On your ear, gently hold where your narrow and wide ridges meet.

Hunger

Did you know reflexology can help curb your cravings? The appetite control point in your ears is especially good at reducing your hunger. First reflex all along the arch of your left foot, move to the soft palm of your left hand, and finish by holding the appetite control point on both ears until your hunger goes away.

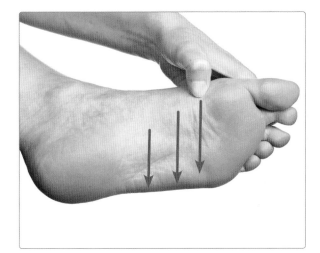

Reflex the arch of your left foot.

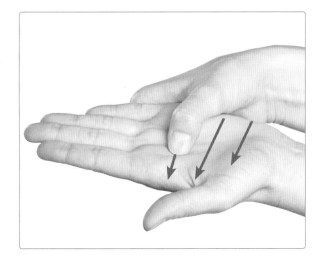

On your left hand, work on the soft part of your palm.

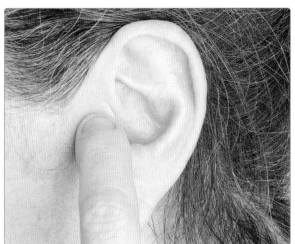

Hold the appetite control point on your ear's facial ridge.

Hypoglycemia

Hypoglycemia occurs when the amount of sugar (glucose) in your blood falls to very low levels. By releasing insulin, your pancreas can help get your blood sugar back in balance. Although the head of your pancreas is on your right side, most of the rest of it is on your left, behind your stomach. So spend most of your time reflexing your left foot, hand, and ear.

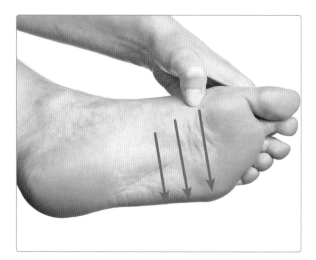

Reflex the arch of your left foot, and spend a little time on your right foot, too.

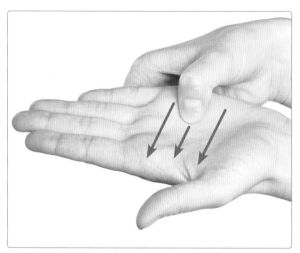

Work on the soft part of the palm of your left hand and also a little on your right hand.

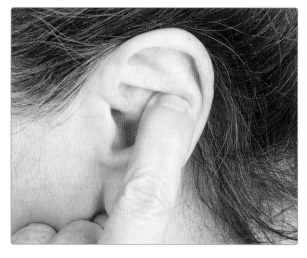

Hold the beginning of the upper valley on your left ear and then move to your right ear.

Immunity

Your immune system does so much within your body to promote good health, and you can help boost its benefits. By reflexing for everything between the top of your neck and your lower abdomen, you'll cover reflexes for many components of your immune system—your thymus, spleen, digestive tract, and appendix as well as lymph nodes through-out your body.

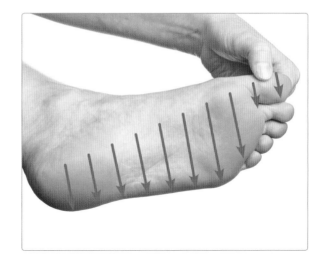

Reflex your big toe, the ball of your foot, your arch, and your heel.

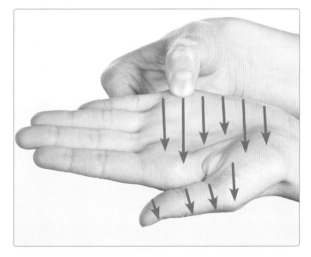

Reflex your thumb, the big knuckles at the base of your fingers, the soft part of your palm, and heel of your hand.

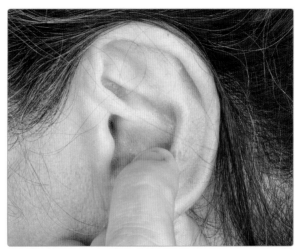

On your ear, reflex halfway up your middle ridge.

Inflammation

Your body naturally produces some inflammation, to use, for example, to help your body heal when you're injured. But excess inflammation can be a problem. To help keep inflammation in balance, your adrenal glands produce adrenocorticosteroids, your body's natural anti-inflammatory chemicals. To relax your adrenal glands so they can better produce these chemicals, spend more of your time reflexing on your feet and hands before moving to your ears and holding your facial ridge.

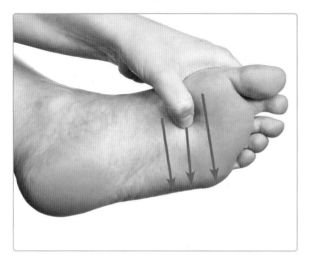

Reflex the upper area of the arch of your foot.

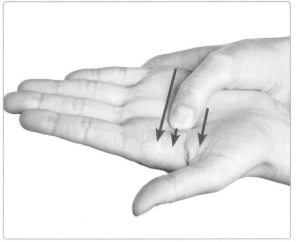

Work the upper area of the soft part of the palm of your hand.

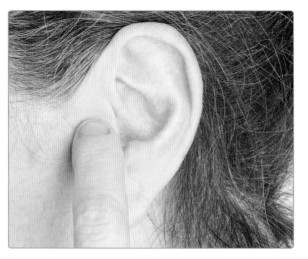

On your ear, hold your facial ridge.

Inner Ear Issues

Inner ear issues can range from balance problems and dizziness to hearing impairment. For relief of symptoms associated with inner ear problems, spend some time working on the middle and inner ear reflexes in your hand, move to the middle and inner ear reflexes in your foot, and finish by holding the middle and inner ear reflex in your earlobe.

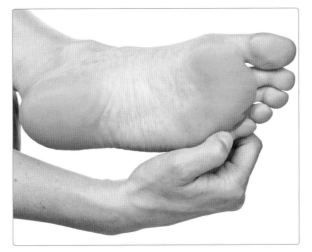

Work on the ridge where the base of your two outermost toes connect to the pad of your foot.

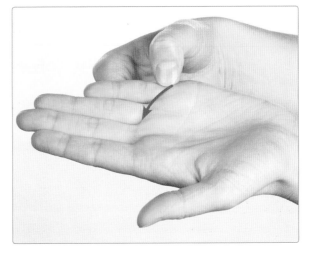

Reflex the ridge where the base of your two outermost fingers connect to the palm of your hand.

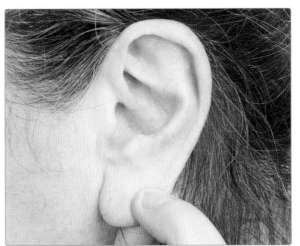

On your ear, reflex slightly back of the middle part of your earlobe.

Intestinal Issues

Whatever type of large or small intestinal issue is troubling you, reflexology can provide some relief. Because your small and large intestines are close together, you can work on reflexes for them both at the same time. Start with your feet first, move to your hands, and finish by firmly working on your ears.

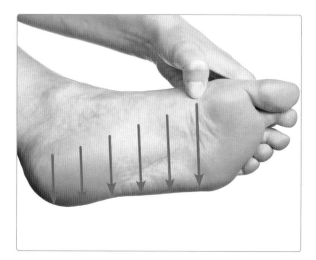

Reflex your arch and the heel of your foot.

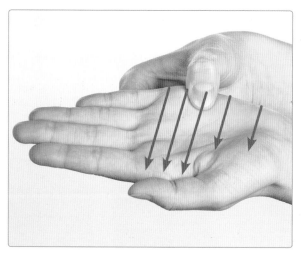

Work on the soft part of your palm and the heel of your hand.

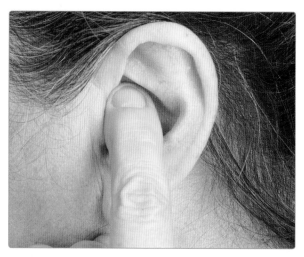

On your ear, reflex your upper valley.

Irregularity

When you're suffering from irregularity, you want to be regular again as soon as you can. Reflexing the arch and heel of your foot, as well as the palm and heel of your hand, can be helpful to return regularity to bowel movements. Work gently, for long periods of time, for best results.

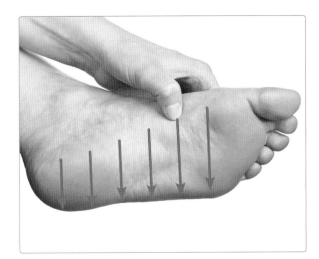

On your foot, reflex your arch and heel.

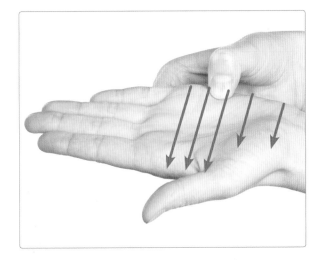

Work on the soft part of the palm of your hand as well as the heel.

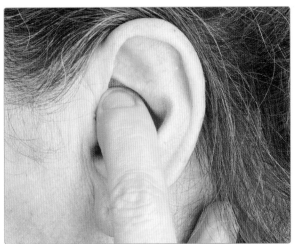

On your ear, hold the upper valley.

Irritability

When you're irritated, it sometimes seems like nothing goes right. For relief of irritability, work on your feet and hands using the entire pad of your thumb. Then, on your ears, hold the tranquilizer point.

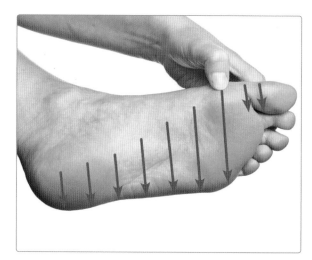

Reflex the base of your big toe and the pad and arch of your foot.

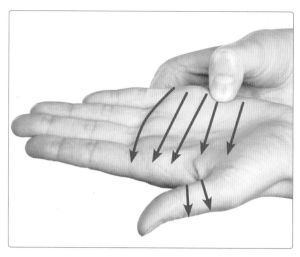

Work along the palm side of your thumb, the knuckles where your fingers join your hand, and the soft part of your palm.

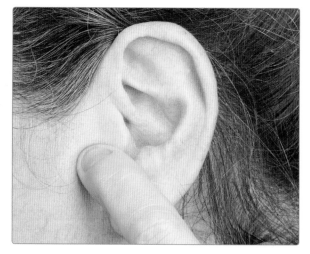

Gently hold your ear's tranquilizer point.

Irritable Bowel Syndrome (IBS)

Irritable bowel syndrome can cause abdominal pain, cramps, bloating, and other uncomfortable symptoms. Gently reflexing the arch and heel of your foot and the palm and heel of your hand can be helpful to reduce bowel pain and discomforts. You can do this work for long periods of time if necessary.

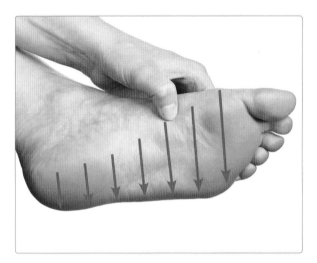

Reflex the arch and heel of your foot.

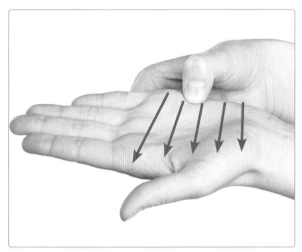

Gently work the soft part of your palm and the heel of your hand.

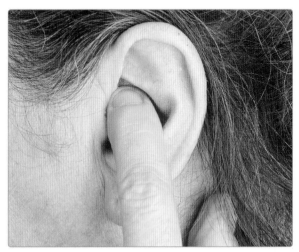

On your ear, reflex your upper valley.

Jaw Pain

Jaw pain can manifest in the joint itself or spread up into your head as well as down into your neck. For more immediate relief of jaw pain, hold the temporomandibular joint (TMJ) point in your ear. For more long-term jaw pain prevention, work on the bottom of your big toe and the palm-side surface of your thumb.

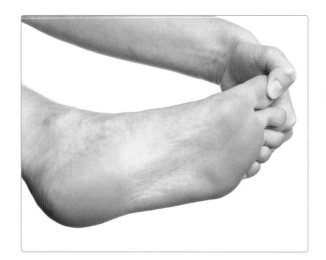

Reflex the bottom surface of the outer half of your big toe.

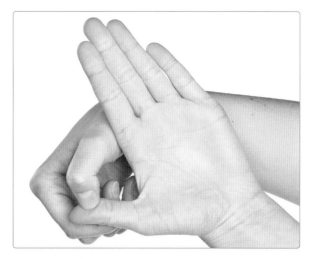

Work on the palm-side surface of the outer half of your thumb.

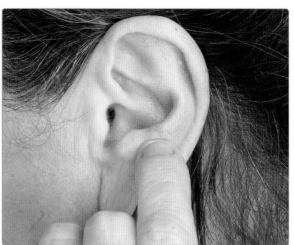

On your ear, reflex the indentation at the base of your outer valley (your TMJ point).

Kidney Infection

For relief of the abdominal pain, fever, and other discomforts that come with a kidney infection, spend some time reflexing the arch of your foot and the soft part of the palm of your hand. Then, in your ear, hold the kidney reflex against your head with the bony tip of your index finger.

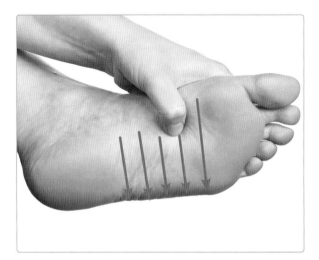

Reflex all over the arch of your foot.

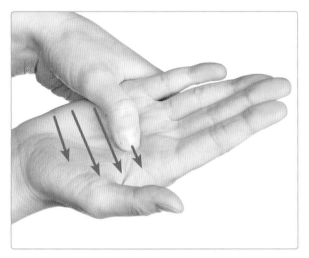

Work all over the soft part of the palm of your hand.

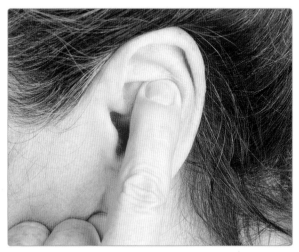

Halfway up the upper valley, hold the kidney reflex using the tip of your index finger.

Kidney Stone

Kidney stones are small balls of mineralized crystals and acid salt that can form anywhere in your urinary tract, from your kidneys to your bladder, and cause intense pain. For relief, reflex the arch of your foot and the soft part of the palm of your hand. Then move to your ear and hold the kidney reflex against your head with the bony tip of your index finger.

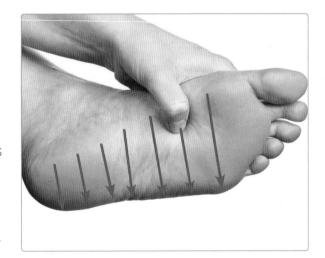

Work all over the arch of your foot and your heel.

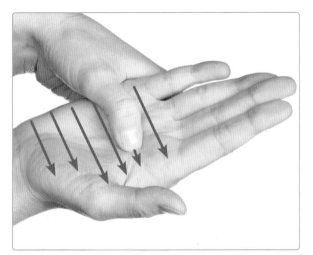

Reflex the soft part of your palm and the heel of your hand.

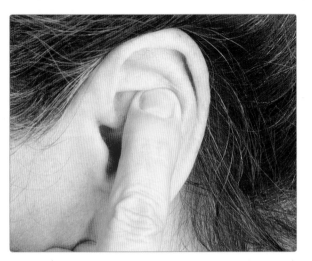

On your ear, reflex the upper half of the upper valley.

Knee Pain

Knee pain can be caused by a number of issues. For relief of the pain and discomfort associated with this joint, spend more time thumb rolling the area in front of and below your outer ankle. Move to your hand and then hold the knee reflex in your ear.

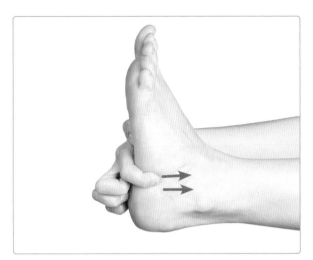

Reflex the outer edge of your foot, below and in front of your ankle bone.

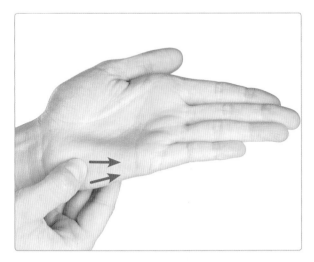

Work on the outer edge of your hand, near your wrist.

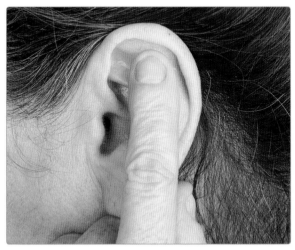

On your ear, hold halfway up the wide ridge.

Leg Cramp

Leg cramps can be brought on by a number of things, and they can occur in almost anyone. For relief, spend more time thumb rolling the area in front of and below your outer ankle, progress to your hand, and finish by holding the leg reflex in your ear.

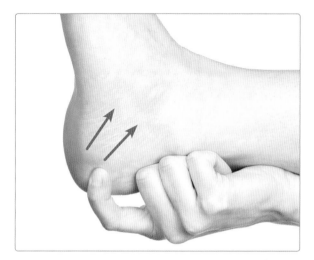

Reflex the outer edge of your foot, below and in front of your ankle bone.

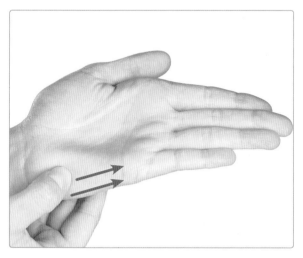

Work the outer edge of your hand, near your wrist.

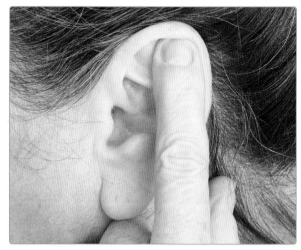

On your ear, hold your wide ridge.

Liver

Your liver does so many jobs. It cleans your blood, houses vitamins, helps with digestion, and much more. To promote good liver health, spend some time reflexing your right foot, hand, and ear—your liver is mostly on the right side of your upper abdomen.

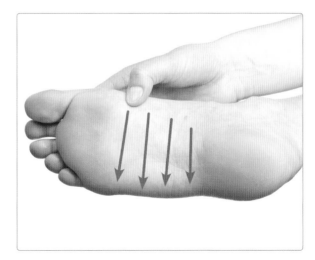

Work on the arch of your right foot and then a little of your left arch.

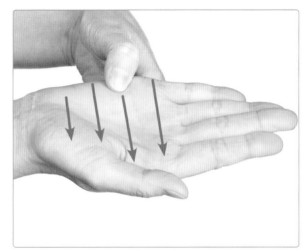

Reflex the soft part of the palm of your right hand and then a little of your left hand.

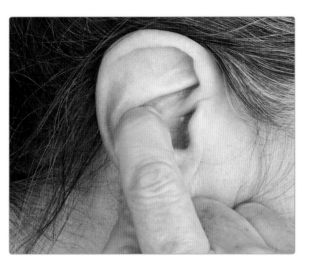

On your right ear, reflex the middle ridge.

Lungs

Your lungs are essential to your good health, and reflexology can help give them a beneficial boost. Spend a lot of time working on the lung reflexes in the grooves in the top of your foot as well as the grooves on the back of your hand. Finish by holding your index finger in the lower valley of your ear.

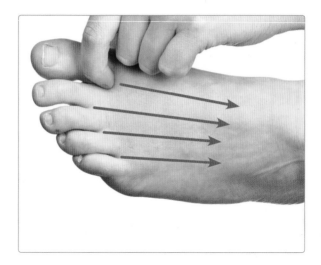

Reflex the grooves on the top of your foot.

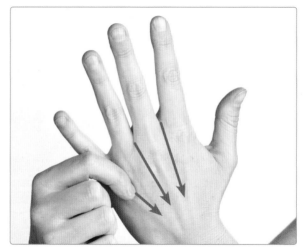

Work on the grooves on the back of your hand.

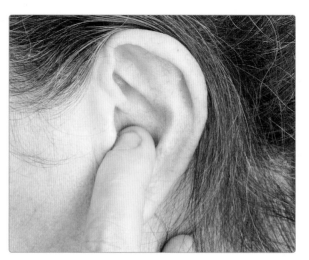

On your ear, hold the center part of your lower valley.

Migraine

Migraines can be debili-
tating and painful. It can
take working on the brain
reflexes for more than
an hour for a migraine to
begin to dissipate. Give
most of your attention to
the brain reflex on your upper earlobe for the fastest
relief.

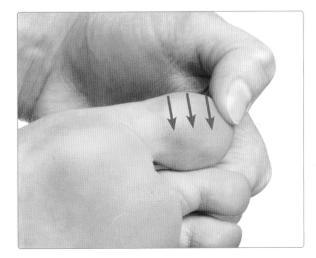

Reflex the
outer half of
the bottom
side of your
big toe.

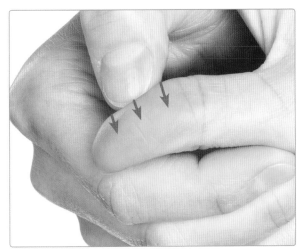

Work on the
outer half of
the palm-side
surface of your
thumb.

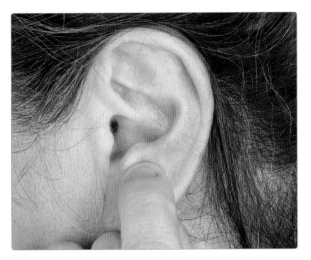

On your ear,
reflex the
upper center of
your earlobe.

Motion Sickness

Motion sickness is triggered by movements that are unfamiliar to your middle and inner ear, and the result is felt in the stomach in the form of nausea and queasiness. For relief, reflex for the stomach and then for the middle and inner ear.

To reflex for your stomach:

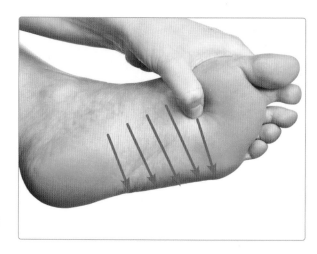

Reflex the arch of your left foot.

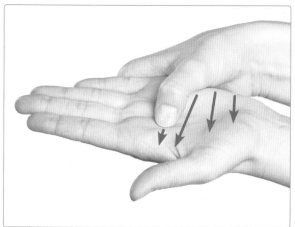

Work on the soft part of the palm of your left hand.

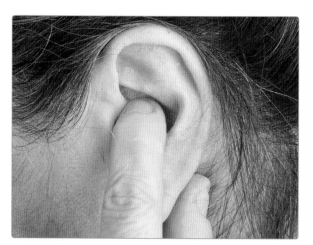

On your left ear, work the middle ridge, near the root of the outer ridge.

To reflex for your middle and inner ear:

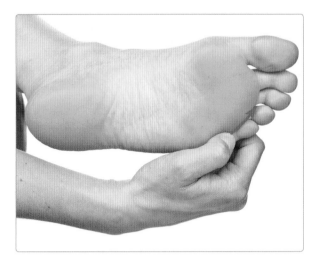

Work on the ridge where the base of your two outermost toes connect to the pad of your foot.

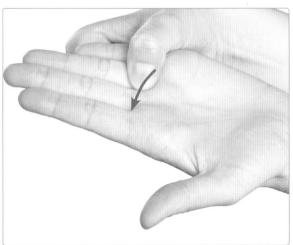

Reflex the ridge where the base of your middle and ring fingers connect to the palm of your hand.

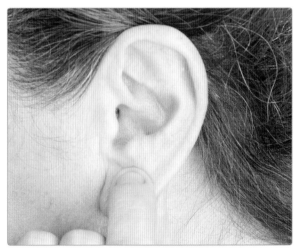

On your ear, reflex slightly back of the middle part of your earlobe.

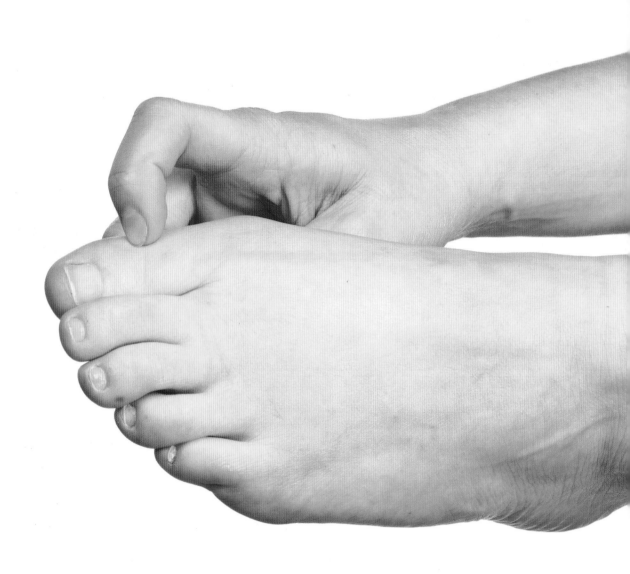

Nausea

When you're feeling nauseated, you want relief fast. Reflex all of the arch of your left foot, and reflex all of the soft part of the palm of your left hand—these two spots are equally effective for relief of nausea. Then, hold the stomach reflex on your left ear.

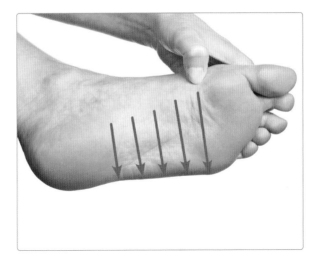

Work on the entire arch of your left foot.

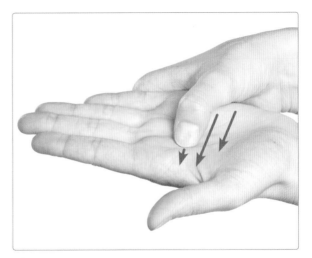

Work all over the soft part of the palm of your left hand.

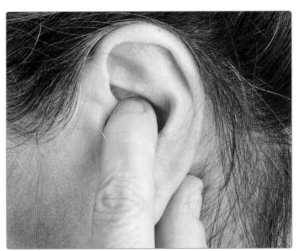

On your left ear, reflex the inner ridge near the root of the outer ridge.

Neck Pain

Neck pain is a common issue among people of all ages. Holding the lower part of the middle ridge in your ear for 10 minutes or more can bring dramatic relief of neck pain. Also work the neck reflexes on your foot and hand.

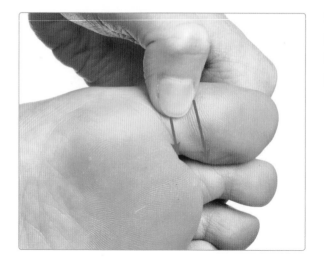

Work on the lower half of the base of your big toe.

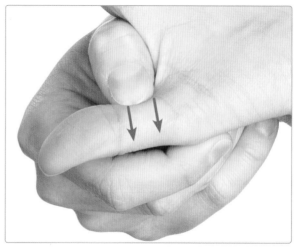

Reflex the bottom half of the palm-side surface of your thumb.

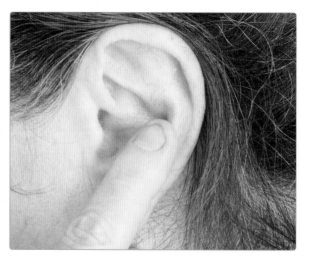

On your ear, hold the lower 1 inch (2.5cm) of your middle ridge.

Pink Eye Discomfort

Reflexology can help dissipate some of the irritation pink eye, or conjunctivitis, can cause. Work primarily on the eye reflexes on the hands at base of your index and middle fingers. Then work the same reflexes on your foot. Finish by holding the eye reflex in your earlobe.

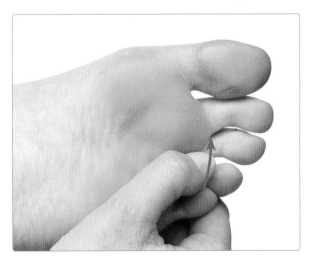

Reflex the ridge where the base of toes 2 and 3 connect to the pad of your foot.

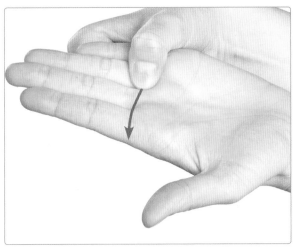

Work on the ridge where the base of your index and middle fingers connect to the palm of your hand.

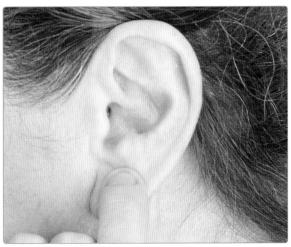

On your ear, hold the middle of your earlobe.

Pneumonia

Pneumonia can cause difficulty breathing, cough, fever, and more. For relief, spend a lot of time working on the lung reflexes in the grooves on the top of your foot and then move to the grooves on the back of your hand. Finish by holding, using your index finger, in your ear's lower valley.

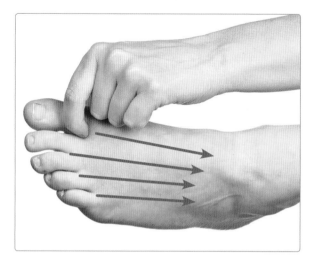

Reflex the grooves on the top of your foot.

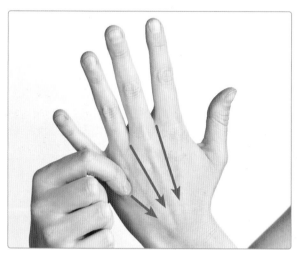

Work on the grooves on the back of your hand.

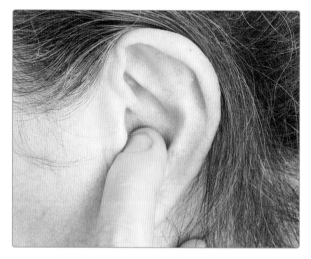

On your ear, reflex the center of your lower valley.

Prostate Problems

Many men live with prostate issues, including an enlarged prostate. When reflexing, spend the majority of your time thumb rolling the area below your inner ankle, move to your hand, and then hold the prostate reflex on your ear.

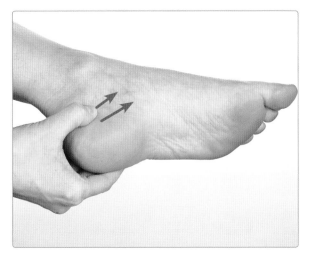

Thumb roll along the inner edge of your foot, below your ankle.

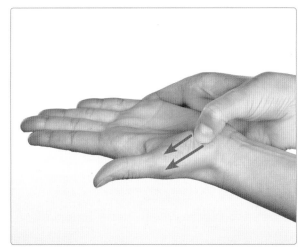

On your hand, reflex the inner edge near your wrist.

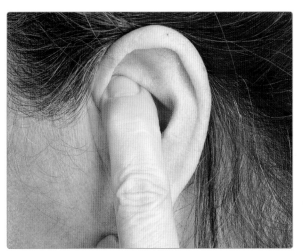

Reflex the uppermost part of the upper valley of your ear.

Psoriasis

Psoriasis is a chronic skin disorder that can cause dry, itchy, red areas anywhere on your body. You can target where you reflex for specific relief, or you can reflex for everything. Avoid reflexing on any skin that is currently inflamed with psoriasis.

If you have psoriasis on your head:

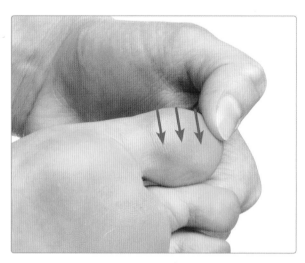

Reflex the outer half of the bottom side of your big toe.

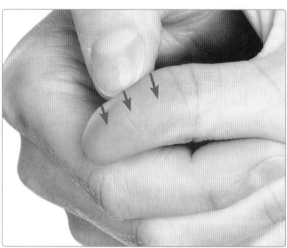

Work on the outer half of the palm-side surface of your thumb.

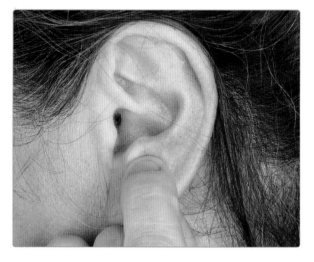

On your ear, gently work on your upper earlobe.

If you have psoriasis on your neck:

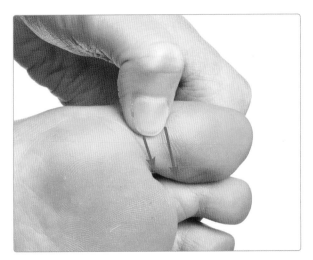

Work on the base of your big toe closest to the pad of your foot.

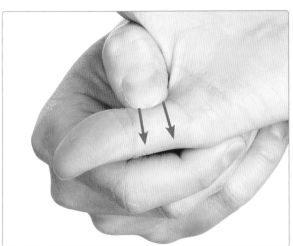

On your hand, work on the lower half of the palm-side surface of your thumb.

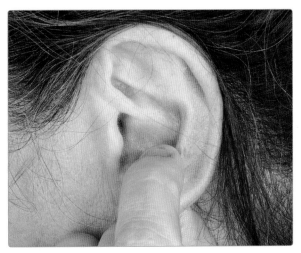

Gently hold the lower 1 inch (2.5cm) of the middle ridge in your ear.

Psoriasis *(continued)*

If you have psoriasis on your chest:

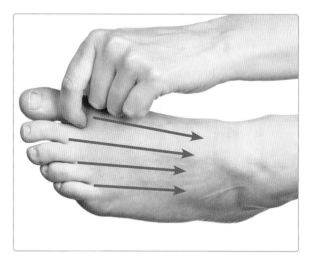

Reflex the grooves on the top of your foot.

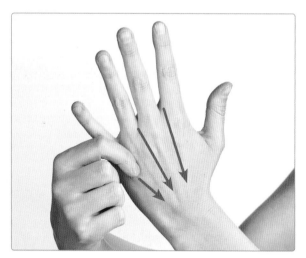

On your hand, work on the grooves on the back of your hand.

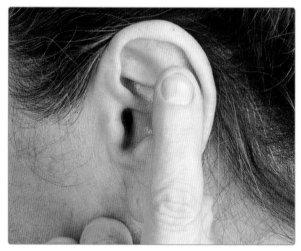

Gently hold the body of the middle ridge in your ear.

If you have psoriasis on your back:

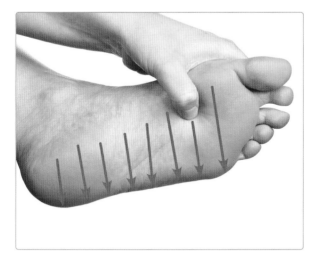

Reflex the inner edge, the arch, and the heel of your foot.

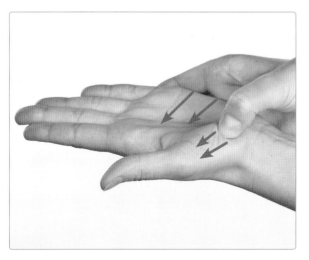

Work all along the inner edge of your hand, plus the palm and the heel.

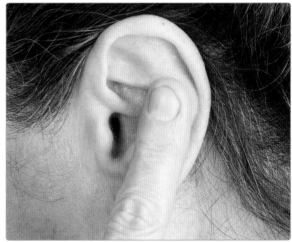

On your ear, reflex the middle ridge.

Psoriasis *(continued)*

If you have psoriasis on your arms:

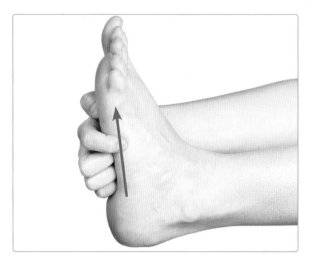

Reflex all along
the outer edge
of your foot.

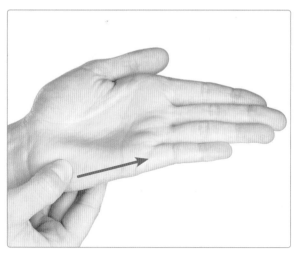

Work all along the outer edge of your hand.

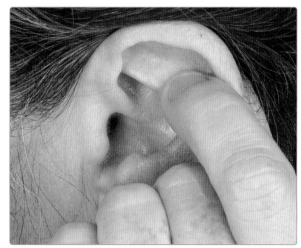

On your ear, gently reflex halfway up the outer valley.

If you have psoriasis on your legs:

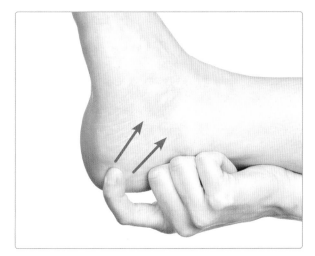

Work on the outer edge of your foot, below and in front of your ankle bone.

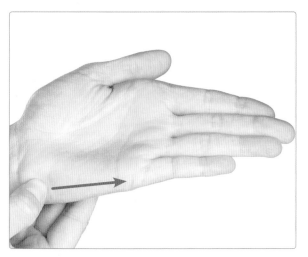

On your hand, reflex the outer edge, near your wrist.

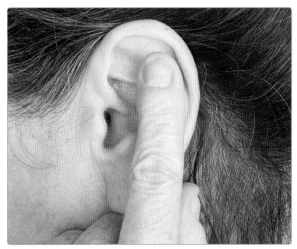

On your ear, reflex the wide ridge.

Ringing in the Ears (Tinnitus)

Reflexology likely won't cure tinnitus, but it could help some. Spend more of your time reflexing the middle and inner ear reflexes on your hand. Then, go to your foot before moving to your ear to hold the middle and inner ear reflex on your earlobe.

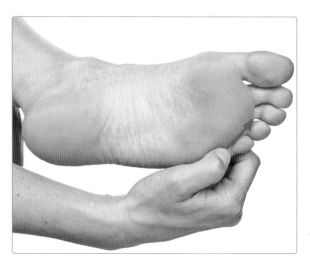

Reflex the ridge where the base of your two outermost toes connect to bottom of your foot.

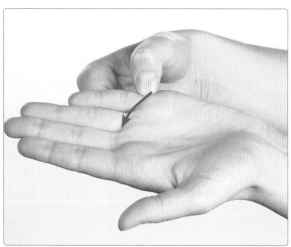

Work on the ridge where the base of your ring and little fingers connect to the palm of your hand.

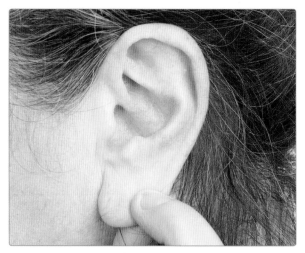

On your ear, gently reflex slightly back of the middle part of your earlobe.

Sciatic Nerve Pain

Your sciatic nerve runs from your lower middle back, through your hips, and down each leg. Sciatica refers to the pain that can pulse all along this nerve. Holding the narrow ridge on your ear for 10, 20, or even 30 minutes can provide amazing relief from sciatic pain. Also work on the sciatic reflexes on your foot and hand.

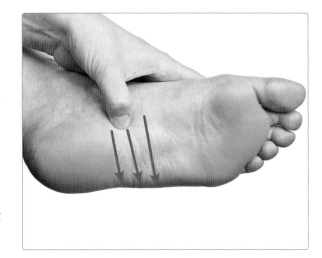

On your foot, work on the area between your arch and your heel.

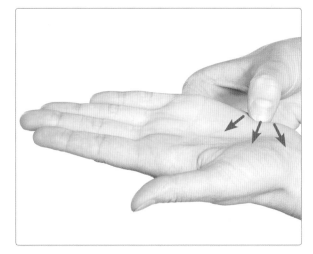

Reflex the area between the soft part of your palm and the heel of your hand.

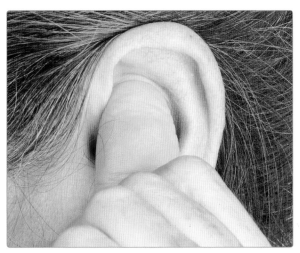

On your ear, firmly hold your narrow ridge.

Scoliosis

When viewed from behind, your spine should be in a straight, vertical line. Scoliosis, an abnormal sideways curve to the spine, sometimes shows up in teen years, but it more commonly occurs later in life. Working the middle part of the inner edge of your foot can be especially helpful for easing scoliosis-related discomfort.

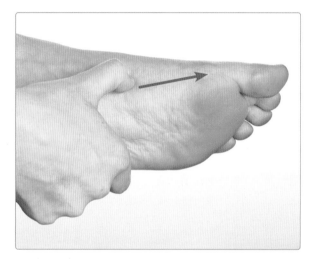

On your foot, reflex midway along the inner edge.

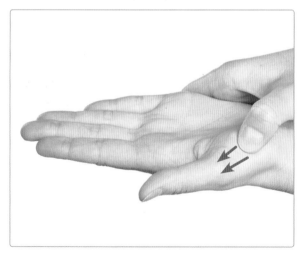

Reflex midway along the inner edge of your hand.

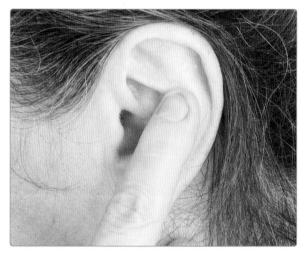

On your ear, reflex midway up the middle ridge.

Seasonal Affective Disorder (SAD)

Especially during winter months, people can sometimes experience seasonal affective disorder, when they feel a bit blue, a bit blah, a bit depressed. Spending lots of time gently reflexing the outer half of your toes and fingers and holding the pineal reflex on your earlobe can help.

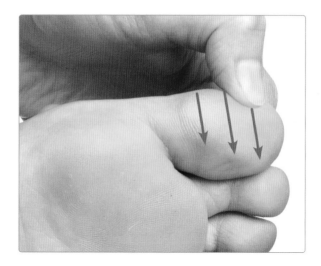

Work on the bottom of your big toe.

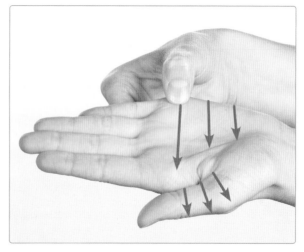

Reflex your palm and the palm-side surface of your thumb.

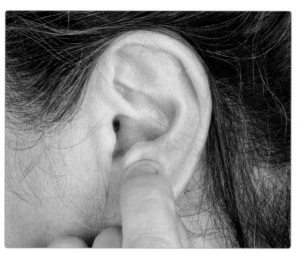

On your ear, hold your earlobe.

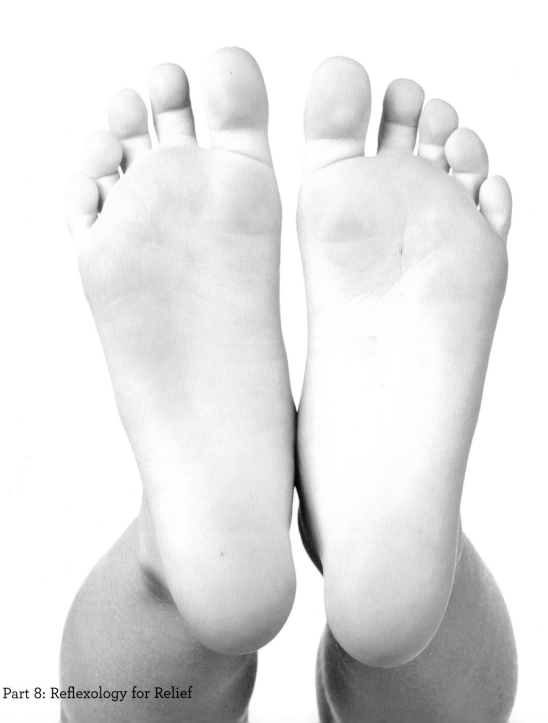

Shin Splints

Shin splints manifest as pain along your shin bone in your leg and often slow down runners. For relief, spend time thumb rolling the area in front of and below your outer ankle. Move to your hand and then hold the lower leg reflex in your ear.

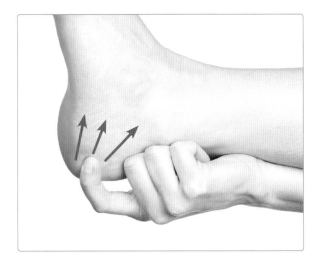

Reflex the outer edge of your foot, below your ankle bone.

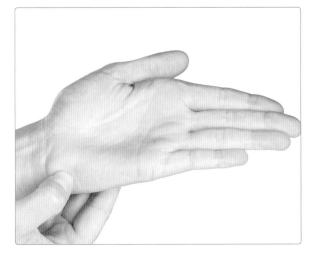

On your hand, reflex the outer edge, near your wrist.

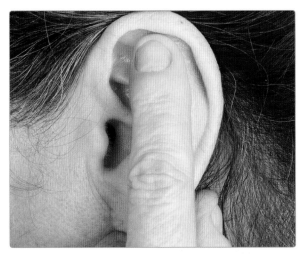

On your ear, gently reflex the upper half of your wide ridge.

Shoulder Pain

Shoulder pain can happen to nearly any one at any age and be the result of a variety of issues. For relief, hold slightly above the base of your ear's middle ridge, outer valley, and outer ridge with the pad of your thumb and index finger. Then reflex the indicated grooves on your foot and hand.

If you have pain in your shoulder joint:

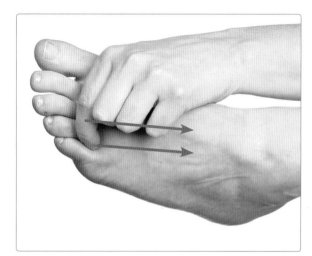

Reflex grooves 4 and 5 on the top of your foot.

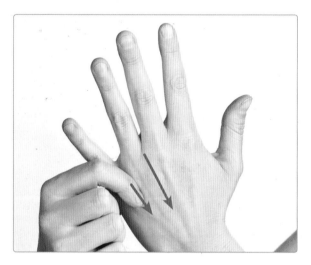

On the back of your hand, reflex grooves 4 and 5.

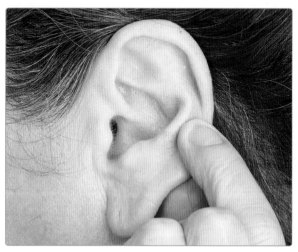

On your ear, hold near the bottom of the outer valley.

If you have pain in the muscles on top of your shoulder:

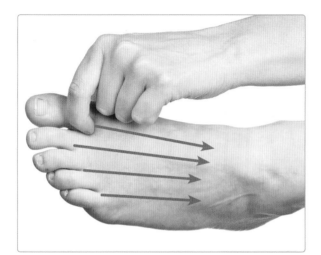

Reflex the webs at the base of your toes.

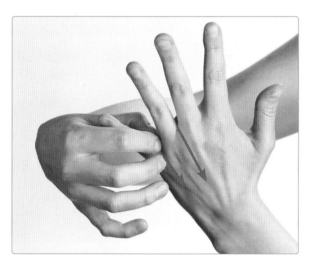

On the back of your hand, reflex grooves 4 and 5.

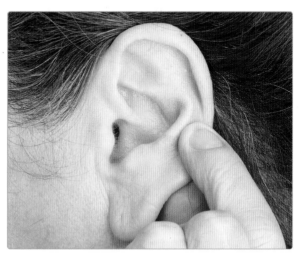

Hold near the bottom of your ear's outer valley.

Shoulder Pain *(continued)*

If you have pain in the muscle between your shoulder blades:

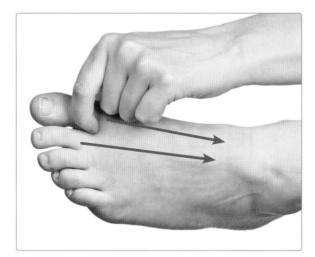

Reflex grooves
1 and 2 on the
top of your
foot.

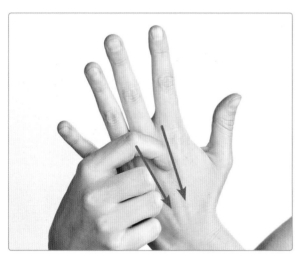

Work on grooves 1 and 2 on the back of your hand.

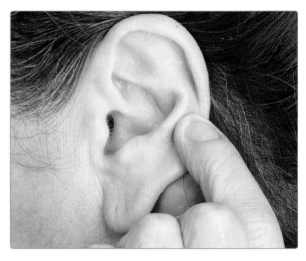

Hold near the bottom of the outer valley on your ear.

If you have pain in your shoulder blades:

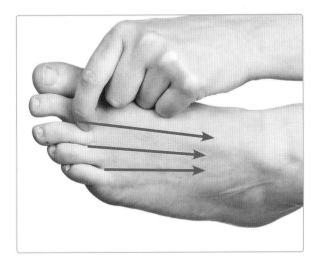

On the top of your foot, work on grooves 2, 3, and 4.

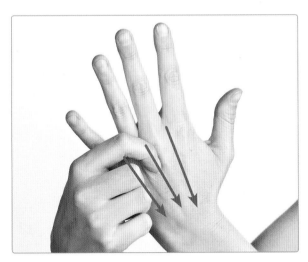

Reflex grooves 2, 3, and 4 on the back of your hand.

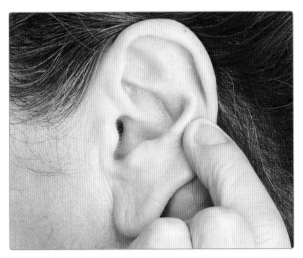

On your ear, hold near the bottom of your outer valley.

Sinus Issues

Sinus issues can range from congestion to a headache—all of it annoying and uncomfortable. For relief, hold the sinus reflex just below the notch ridge in your earlobe. Then move to the three soft sides of your toes, and finish by working on the three soft sides of your fingers.

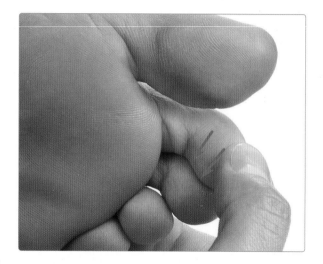

Reflex the three soft sides of each of your toes.

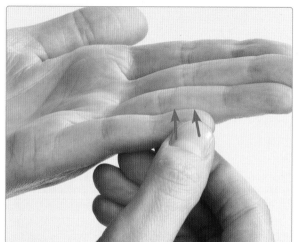

On your hand, reflex the three soft sides of your thumb and fingers.

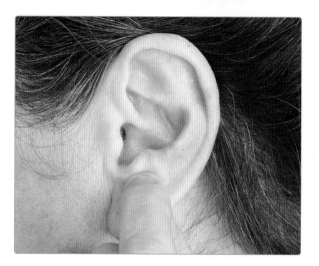

Hold the upper part of your earlobe, near the notch ridge.

Sore Throat

For a sore throat, work the neck reflexes on your foot and hand. Also spend some time reflexing your ears, pushing on the throat reflex with the tip of your index finger.

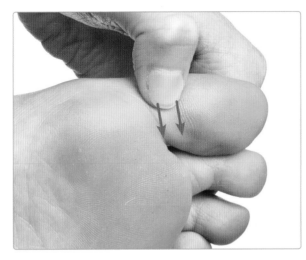

Reflex the lower half of the bottom side of your big toe.

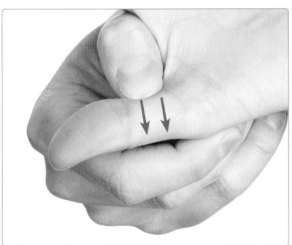

Reflex the bottom half of the palm-side surface of your thumb.

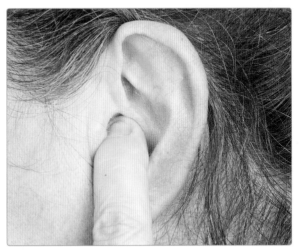

On your ear, reflex the upper part of your lower valley, near your ear canal.

Stomachache

Stomach upset can be caused by a number of issues. For relief, reflex all of the arch on your left foot and all of the soft part of the palm of your left hand. Then, hold the stomach reflex on your left ear.

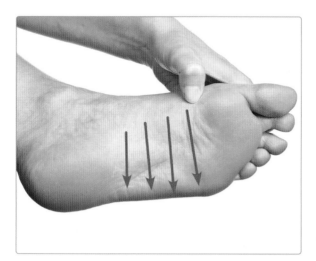

Reflex all over the arch of your left foot.

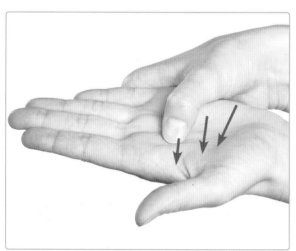

On your left hand, work on the soft part of your palm.

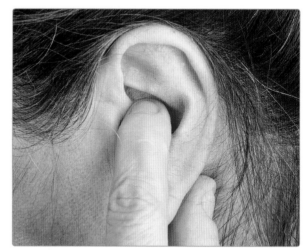

On your left ear, reflex the middle ridge near the base of the outer ridge.

Stress

Few people do not experience some level of stress from time to time. To help combat the tense feelings stress can bring, squeeze the area above your earlobe, near your face, between your thumb and index finger and flow down slowly. Repeat for a minute or two before moving on to reflex your foot and hand.

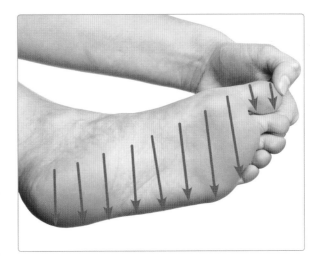

Reflex the bottom side of your big toe and the bottom of your foot.

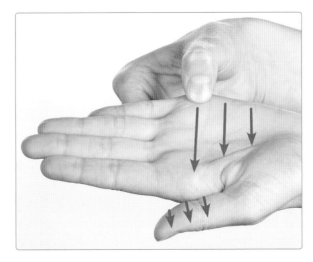

On your hand, work your palm and the palm-side surface of your thumb.

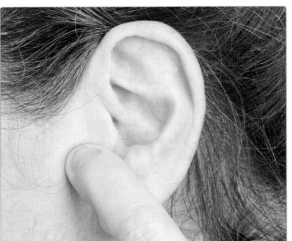

On your ear, reflex the tranquilizer point between your notch ridge and your face.

Temporomandibular Joint (TMJ) Disorder

Temporomandibular joint disorder can mean pain in the muscles and joint of the jaw. For more immediate relief of jaw pain, hold the TMJ point in your ear. For more long-term relief, and to reduce the incidents of recurrence, work on the bottom of your big toe and the palm-side surface of your thumb.

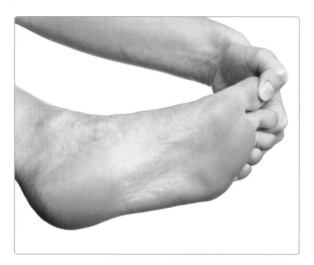

Reflex the bottom, outer half of your big toe.

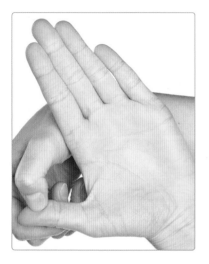

Reflex the palm-side surface of the outer half of your thumb.

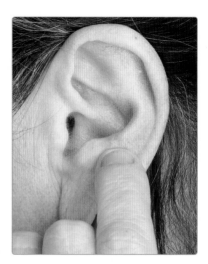

On your ear, reflex the indentation at the base of the outer valley.

Thyroid

Your thyroid is a gland located at the bottom of your neck that helps regulate many functions in your body. For thyroid health, work the lower neck reflexes on your foot and hand. On your ear, hold the thyroid reflex, about 1 inch (2.5cm) above base of the middle ridge.

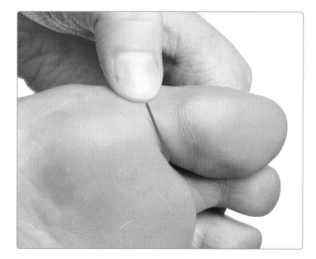

On your foot, reflex all around the base of your big toe.

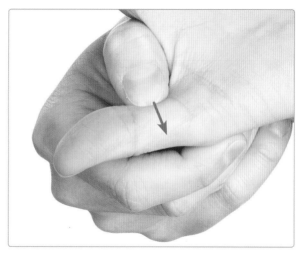

Work all around the base of your thumb.

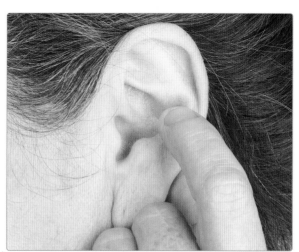

On your ear, reflex about one third of the way up the middle ridge.

Tonsillitis

Tonsillitis is the inflammation of your tonsils, which are located in the back of your mouth, at the top of your throat. For relief of the sore throat, difficulty swallowing, and other symptoms of tonsillitis, in addition to working your big toe and thumb, hold the tonsil reflex near the bottom of your earlobe.

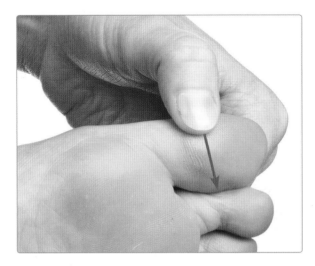

Work on the middle third of the bottom side of your big toe.

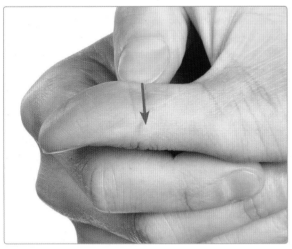

On your hand, reflex the middle third of the palm-side surface of your thumb.

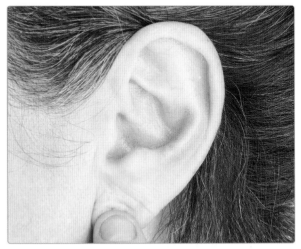

Hold the middle part of your lower earlobe.

Toothache

If you have a toothache, you likely need to see your dentist. To relieve the pain and discomfort in the meantime, reflexology can help. The bony knuckles of your feet and hands can be especially tender, so start with a flatter thumb roll, gradually using more of the tip of your thumb.

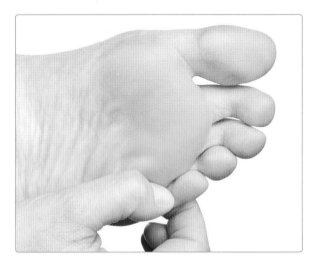

Reflex the bottom side of the middle knuckle of each toe.

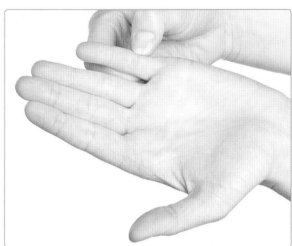

On your hand, reflex the palm-side surface of each finger's middle knuckle.

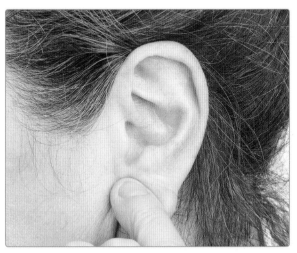

Work your upper earlobe, near your face.

Ulcer

The pain and burning of an ulcer is hard to ignore. Reflexology can offer some relief of the symptoms of gastric and duodenal ulcers. For a gastric ulcer, focus on the arch of your left foot and the soft part of the palm of your left hand. These areas are equally effective at relieving stomach ulcer pain. Be sure to hold the stomach reflex on your left ear, too. Because your duodenum is in your right mid abdomen, work on your right foot, hand, and ear, spending extra time reflexing the arch of your foot and the soft part of your palm.

If you have a gastric ulcer:

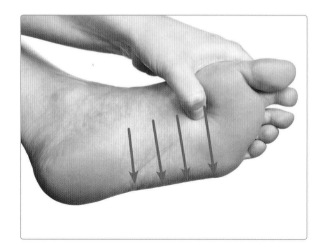

On your left foot, work all over your arch.

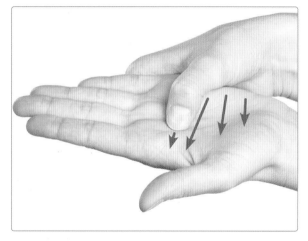

Work on the soft part of the palm of your left hand.

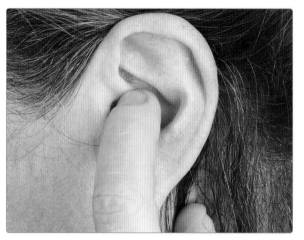

On your left ear, reflex the middle ridge near root of the outer ridge.

If you have a duodenal ulcer:

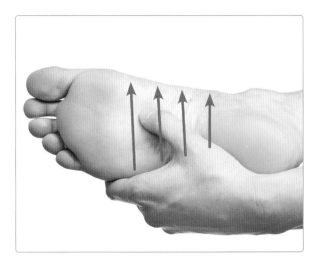

Reflex the arch of your right foot.

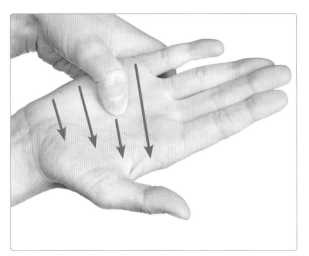

On your right hand, work on the soft part of your palm.

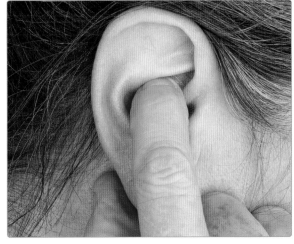

Gently reflex the lower part of the upper valley of your right ear.

Urinary Tract Infection (UTI)

A urinary tract infection can occur anywhere along your urinary tract—and can be painful. Using a high thumb roll on your foot's urinary bladder reflex can ease UTI pain. Repeat several times a day, for about 10 minutes each time.

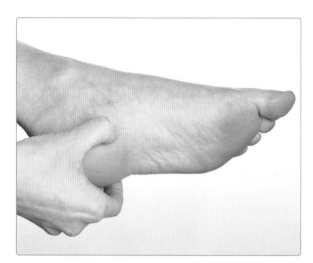

Reflex the inner edge of your foot near where your arch and heel meet.

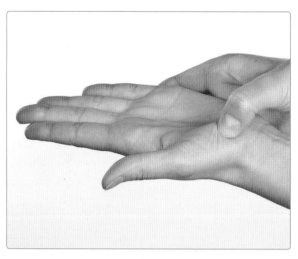

On your hand, work on the inner edge, near your wrist.

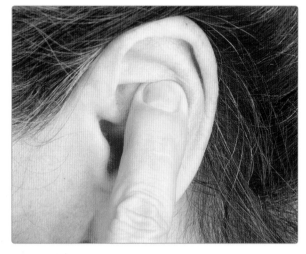

Reflex the upper part of the upper valley of your ear.

Vomiting

Vomiting can be the result of a number of different issues, from the morning sickness pregnant women sometimes experience to something you ate or drank upsetting your stomach. For relief, work all over the arch of your left foot and all over the soft part of your left palm. Both are equally effective for relaxing upper abdominal muscles. Then finish by holding the stomach reflex on your left ear.

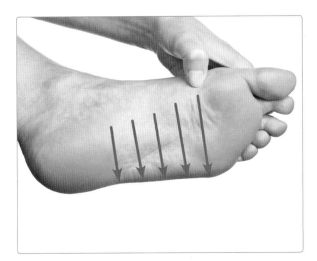

Reflex all over the arch of your left foot.

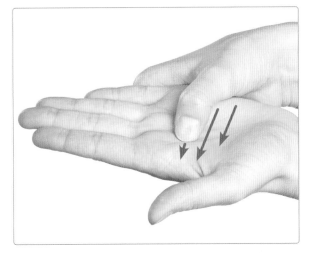

On your left hand, work all over the soft part of your palm.

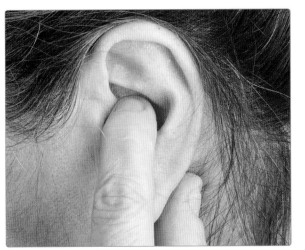

Hold the middle ridge near the base of the outer ridge on your left ear.

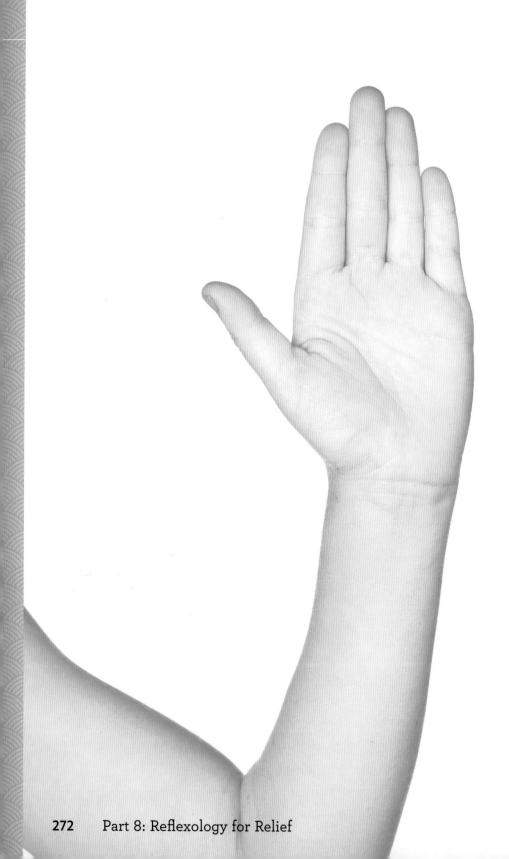

Wrist Pain

You use your hands for so much during your day, having wrist pain can put a damper on your movement. For relief, work on your wrist reflex on the outer edge of your hand for quite awhile. Then progress to the wrist reflex on your foot, and finish with some work on your ear's wrist reflex.

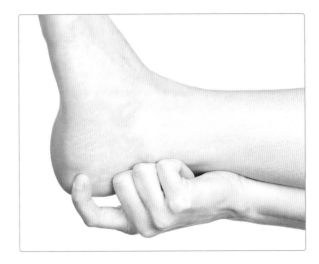

Reflex the outer edge of your foot, below your ankle bone.

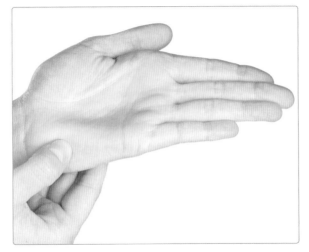

Reflex the outer edge of your hand, near your wrist.

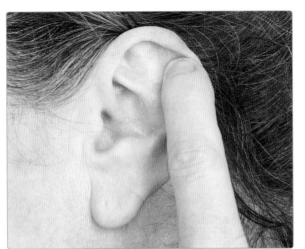

On your ear, reflex near the top of the outer valley.

Glossary

allergy point   A reflex at the top of your ear that helps reduce or eliminate allergic symptoms and reactions when worked.

antidepression point   A reflex near the top of your earlobe that helps with easing depression-related feelings when worked.

anxiety point   A reflex near the bottom of your earlobe that helps soothe your body when worked.

appetite control point   A reflex on the flap of your ear that protects your ear canal and helps reduce hunger and food cravings when worked.

chart   *See* reflex map.

detoxification   The process of your body ridding itself of toxins accumulated from the air, food and drink, and the environment as a whole—in addition to waste products produced as a result of your body's cells using oxygen and nutrients—via your circulatory and lymphatic systems. If done too quickly, detoxification can cause itchiness, nausea, headaches, irritability, and sluggishness. Although such reactions are not common, it's often recommended to drink plenty of extra water after reflexology sessions to help minimize or prevent these possible detoxification reactions.

ear reflexology   The act of using unique nurturing touch techniques on the reflexes on the outer ears.

endocrine point   A reflex found on the top of your ear's notch ridge, the notch between your earlobe and face, that relates to your pituitary gland. It directly affects your other endocrine glands, which in turn impact, directly or indirectly, most functions of your body.

finger roll   A reflexing technique in which you place the pad of your finger on your feet or hands and, while maintaining pressure, roll from the pad of your finger toward the tip. *See also* sideways finger roll; three-finger roll.

flowing   A reflexing technique in which you move your thumbs or fingers very slowly over the surface of the skin to help break down toxins, feel textures on and under the skin, and provide a soothing effect.

foot reflexology   The act of using unique nurturing touch techniques on the reflexes on the feet.

foot roller   *See* roller.

hand reflexology   The act of using unique nurturing touch techniques on the reflexes on the hands.

holding   A reflexing technique in which you place the tip or pad of your fingers or thumbs against parts of your feet, hands, or ears, and maintain still, steady, prolonged pressure.

map   *See* reflex map.

pressure   The depth to which your fingers or thumbs push into the tissue they're touching.

pressure map   *See* reflex map.

reflex   A specific location that, when touched, triggers the body to have a response in a related part of the body. Can also refer to the action of applying pressure with your fingers and thumbs to your feet, hands, or ears.

reflex area   A large surface area on the feet, hands, or ears that corresponds to a large part of the body, such as the shoulders or stomach. *See also* reflex point.

reflex chart   *See* reflex map.

reflex map   An arrangement of reflexes, or pressure points, in a specific design that strongly suggests the shape of the human body. Your feet, hands, and ears all contain specific reflex maps of your body.

reflex point   A small, specific place on the feet, hands, or ears that corresponds to another, small part of the body, such as specific teeth. *See also* reflex area.

reflexing technique   A specific way of using your fingers and thumbs to apply pressure during a reflexology session. Thumb roll, index finger roll, sideways index finger roll, index and middle finger roll, three-finger roll, rotating, holding, flowing, and applying pressure are all specific techniques used in this book.

reflexology roller   *See* roller.

reflexology routine   A session during which you reflex all areas of a part of the body—feet, hands, or ears—in an orderly progression.

relaxation technique   A movement of hands, applied to touching feet, hands, and ears, to help dissipate chemicals from the feet, hands, and ears, to improve circulation, and to have either a soothing or stimulating result.

roller   A reflexology tool, often made of wood or plastic, that can range in size from 6 to 12 inches (15 to 30cm) wide, with a variety of types of ridges, grooves, bumps, and protrusions. It's used to help you apply pressure to reflexology areas and points.

sideways finger roll   A reflexing technique in which you apply pressure with one corner of your index finger and, while maintaining the same level of pressure, roll over the tip of your finger to the other corner of your finger tip. *See also* finger roll.

sleep disorders point   A reflex in the outer valley of your ear that helps you get to sleep and sleep longer and deeper.

temporomandibular joint (TMJ) point   A reflex in the indentation between the bottom of the outer valley of your ear and your earlobe that helps relax jaw muscles when worked and eases or eliminates related pain.

three-finger roll   A reflexing technique in which you place the pad of your index, middle, and ring fingers on your feet or hands and, while maintaining pressure, roll from the pad of your fingers toward the tips. *See also* finger roll; sideways finger roll.

thumb roll   A reflexing technique in which you place the pad of your thumb on your feet or hands and, while maintaining even pressure, roll from the pad of your thumb toward the tip.

tranquilizer point   A reflex between the notch ridge of your ear and your face that helps with relaxation when worked.

zero point   A reflex in the center of your outer ear that can have an impact on the nerve network in back of your upper abdomen, called the celiac ganglion, which can help relax your lower chest and upper and lower abdomen when worked.

Index